Vitamins
& Minerals
HANDBOOK

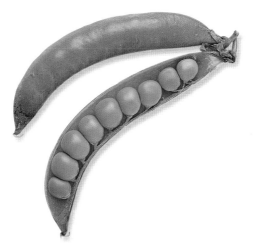

AMANDA URSELL

A Dorling Kindersley Book

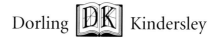
Dorling DK Kindersley

LONDON, NEW YORK, MELBOURNE,
MUNICH AND DELHI

Project Editor Susannah Steel
Art Editor Alison Lotinga
Managing Editor Gillian Roberts
Managing Art Editor Tracey Ward
Category Publisher Mary-Clare Jerram
Art Director Tracy Killick
DTP Designers Louise Paddick and Louise Waller
Production Manager Maryann Webster
US Editor Crystal A. Coble
US Editorial Director LaVonne Carlson

First American Edition 2001
2 4 6 8 10 9 7 5 3 1
Published in the United States by DK Publishing, Inc.,
375 Hudson Street, New York, New York 10014

Library of Congress Cataloging-in-Publication Data

Vitamins and minerals handbook.
        p. cm.
    Includes index.
    ISBN 0-7894-7180-9 (alk. paper)
        1. Vitamins--Popular works. 2. Minerals in human nutrition--
    Popular works. I.Dorling Kindersley Limited.
    QP771 .V57355 2001
    615'.328--dc21   00-045194

Color reproduced by Colourscan, Singapore
Printed and bound in China by South China Printing Co. Ltd

While the author has made every effort to provide accurate and up to date information at
the time of writing, nutritional and medical science is constantly evolving. People should
always consult a qualified medical or dietetic practitioner for individual health advice,
rather than use the general information in this book to treat specific health problems.

see our complete
catalog at
www.dk.com

Contents

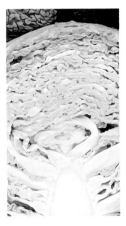
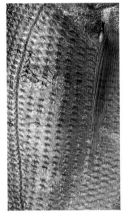
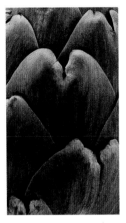

AUTHOR'S INTRODUCTION

In this age, more and more people are becoming interested in improving and maintaining their personal health. To gain optimum physical and mental wellbeing, we must make sure we have the appropriate nutrients our bodies need.

We now realize that our diet plays a significant role in maintaining our health, preventing disease, and, in some cases, maybe even altering the duration or outcome of an illness or chronic condition. These factors have inspired many of us to look more deeply into how best to improve our nutritional status. In many cases, this desire to take responsibility for our own health has led to an increased demand for, an explosion of scientific research into, and the development of effective dietary supplements.

SIGN OF THE TIMES

There is an abundance of different manufactured supplements now readily available from health food stores and pharmacies. While the huge amount of choice can be a potential benefit, the variety of products can often seem too overwhelming and confusing when you are faced by endless rows of bottles and boxes. The contents of these packs can also present us with another choice – whether to choose tablets, capsules, powders, or liquids, and so on. And not only are

there a plethora of vitamins and minerals, which come as single supplements or mixed with each other, but there is also a huge range of products that are based on traditional herbal therapies as a result of the massive resurgence of interest in natural herbal remedies.

We are also experiencing the blossoming of a whole new area of nutrition in the form of "phyto-nutrients" ("phyto" meaning plant). Recent nutritional research into plants has revealed that they can carry beneficial antioxidants, which inhibit the formation of free radicals in the body and therefore may help to improve our general wellbeing and health.

CUTTING THROUGH THE CONFUSION

It is not surprising, therefore, that it is sometimes hard to know where to start when selecting an individual program to benefit our dietary health and vitality.

The *Vitamins and Minerals Handbook* aims to cut through all this confusion and guide you toward choosing the most appropriate supplements according to your age and your general state of health and activity.

WHEN TO THINK ABOUT TAKING SUPPLEMENTS

While a balanced diet and active lifestyle are the bedrock of good health, it is now acknowledged that in certain situations and at different times in our lives there will be extra demands, stresses, and strains that may make the taking of supplements a valid course of action.

Leading a busy lifestyle, eating on the run, consuming an increased number of ready prepared foods, recovering from an illness, planning a pregnancy, eating a vegetarian diet, or simply growing older can all put extra pressure on our bodies.

Add to this scenario the factor that there are some nutrients that may actually be difficult to obtain regularly in adequate quantities from food sources (such as folic acid and vitamin D). In this situation, it is easy to see how regular supplements may be beneficial.

ATTAINING OPTIMAL HEALTH AND VITALITY

There is also a growing school of thought suggesting that, rather than relying on traditional levels of nutrient intakes that help to maintain our health, we should in fact be consuming larger amounts that optimize it. In some instances, there is enough scientific research to suggest this stance is valid, in others we are still awaiting confirmation that it is an appropriate

course of action. The *Vitamins and Minerals Handbook* gives you the opportunity to decide whether to take supplement levels at the Recommended Daily Amount (RDA) or to increase them to Optimal Recommended Intakes. Either way, safe upper levels are provided so that intakes do not become excessive and harmful.

The other important factor that must be taken into account is that if you want to purchase certain supplements but have a specific ailment or condition, you should always consult your doctor first to avoid any confusion. It is possible that some supplements can affect the activity and effectiveness of medical drugs. If you are on or are being put on medication, it is vital that your doctor knows about any other doses you are taking. Finally, if you are at all unsure about your particular situation, then discuss your plans with your doctor first.

You will also find details about when it is best to take individual supplements. Other important factors are mentioned, too, such as what will enhance or decrease the absorption and activity of a vitamin, mineral, or herbal supplement in the body. There is also information outlining any relevant precautions you should be aware of.

Whether you want to dispel any myths, check up on the right kind of supplement intake, or discover which supplement is most suited to helping improve the quality of your health and lifestyle, it is all here in this quick and decisive guide.

WHAT ARE VITAMINS & MINERALS?

Vitamins and minerals are substances that are vital to human health. Without them the body cannot function properly and may become susceptible to a variety of deficiency diseases.

Vitamins must be present in our diets for our bodies to work efficiently and resist illness. Even in the fourth century B.C., physicians such as Hippocrates knew that certain foods prevented particular illnesses. A lack of vitamin C, for example, can eventually lead to scurvy. The only two vitamins that are not derived solely from our diet are vitamins D and K, as they are made, or synthesized, by the body.

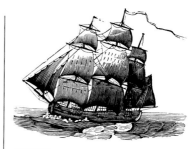

SCURVY
While away at sea for months on end with no fresh fruit or vegetables to eat, many sailors in the 1800s developed scurvy.

THE DISCOVERY OF VITAMINS

It was not until the twentieth century that scientists successfully isolated vitamins from foods and identified their structure. We now know about 13 of these organic substances, all of which are found in food and drink. At its initial discovery, each vitamin was given a letter, for example "A" or "C." Once its chemical structure had been determined, it was then also given a specific name. Vitamin A is therefore also known as retinol, and vitamin C as ascorbic acid. However, like all things, there is the odd exception. Vitamin B, for

example, is not one vitamin but an entire group, and while most of the B-vitamins have their own individual name and number, some, like folate, are known just by their name.

Vitamins are broadly divided into two categories. Those in the first category are needed by the body on a regular basis because they dissolve in water and are quickly lost from the body via the urine. Vitamin C and the B-vitamins are all classified as water-soluble. The remaining vitamins – vitamins A, D, E, and K – are all fat-soluble and belong to the second category. Because these vitamins dissolve in fat, they can remain in the body's fat stores for months or even years.

When you buy vitamin supplements in a health food store or pharmacy, you may find that the label on the bottle sometimes gives the chemical name only. These alternative names are listed under each individual vitamin entry in part one *(pp.26–51)*.

MINERALS

Minerals are inorganic substances that have their origins in non-living things, such as rocks and metal ores. These substances find their way into the food chain by being integrated into the soil in which plants are rooted: we either get our minerals directly by eating these plants, or by eating animals that have previously fed on these plants.

Like vitamins, minerals are needed in small quantities; without them the body cannot function properly. There are 22 minerals that are essential to health. For example, calcium to build strong bones and teeth, and iron to help the brain to concentrate and the body to feel energetic and lively.

Minerals are divided into two main groups:
• Major minerals, such as calcium, magnesium, potassium, chloride, sodium, sulfur, and phosphorus,
• Trace minerals, such as copper, chromium, fluoride, selenium, and zinc, which are needed by the body in smaller quantities.

As with vitamins, a lack of minerals in the diet may cause disease. Conversely, large intakes of certain minerals can also be dangerous, so it is important not to consume too much of a particular mineral, either through diet or by taking too many supplements.

TAKING SUPPLEMENTS

While eating a healthy, balanced diet should supply all the vitamins and minerals most of us need to maintain health and prevent the development of deficiency diseases, there are some groups of people who may need extra help in getting adequate amounts of these essential substances at certain times in their lives:
• Anyone with a busy lifestyle may skip meals and grab snacks instead, which often lack adequate levels of vitamins and minerals.
• Vegetarians, and people on special diets, may not always eat adequate amounts of iron and vitamin B12.
• Pregnant women have increased needs for certain vitamins and minerals.
• As we age, our ability to absorb nutrients effectively decreases, and older people may find it hard to eat well enough to combat this.
• People who frequently play sports and those people who drink and smoke may also have requirements above those normally needed for their sex and age.

In all these cases, a modest supplement may be appropriate. Vitamins and minerals may also have therapeutic properties, helping people to recover more quickly from ill health, and some with antioxidant properties may play a role in helping to prevent diseases such as cancers and heart disease.

OTHER COMMON SUPPLEMENTS

In addition to vitamins and minerals, there are many other supplements available in pharmacies and health stores. These can be broadly divided into two categories: herbal preparations and other nutritional supplements.

HERBAL PREPARATIONS

Herbs have been used in the treatment and prevention of diseases for thousands of years. Each different part of the herb – leaves, roots, bark, stems, flowers, fruit, and seeds – can contain pharmacologically active chemicals. It is these chemicals that determine which part of the plant is used in the preparation of each particular

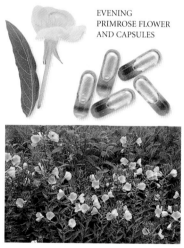

EVENING PRIMROSE FLOWER AND CAPSULES

EVENING PRIMROSE OIL
It takes 5,000 seeds from the evening primrose plant to make one 500mg capsule. The Efamol brand of evening primrose oil is one of the most intensively studied supplements in the world.

remedy. In the case of St. John's wort *(see also p.111)*, for example, the active substance known as hypericin can be found in tiny red sacs on the underside of the plant's leaves. The active chemical silymarin, by comparison, can be detected in extracts of the seeds of the milk thistle plant *(p.107)*.

Herbalists have known for centuries the effect of their herbal preparations on the human body, and have long prescribed a range of remedies such as teas or infusions, tinctures, and decoctions to treat their patients. However, modern science has now made it possible to isolate and standardize extracts so they can be produced as tablets and capsules.

TAKING SENSIBLE PRECAUTIONS

Because herbs are natural substances, there is often a tendency to assume that they are all completely safe to take and can be used by everyone for any purpose. The truth is that herbs can have profound effects on the body's chemistry, and some even have side effects. It is

ECHINACEA
FLOWER
AND
CAPSULES

ECHINACEA PLANT
Also known as the purple
coneflower, native Americans traditionally
used echinacea to treat snakebite and colds.
The plant is widely known for its antiviral
and antibacterial properties, and is still
taken today to treat the common cold.

important not to self-medicate a problem without first seeking advice from your doctor, who can diagnose your condition properly. Once you know the parameters of your particular problem, and you still would like to treat it using herbal preparations, it is best to consult a qualified medical herbalist or pharmacist before purchasing herbal supplements.

OTHER NUTRITIONAL SUBSTANCES

Falling into the category of being neither vitamins, minerals, or herbs, an ever-expanding group of supplements can also be included under the heading of "other nutritional substances." This can incorporate anything from the oil

PRACTITIONER
Many well-known
herbal remedies are now
undergoing scientific
tests, proving to the
medical world that
in some cases they
offer an alternative to
prescription drugs.

pressed from the seeds of the evening primrose plant *(p.98)*, to probiotics *(p.109)*, amino acids, and plant nutrients such as the pigment beta-carotene *(p.91)*, and antioxidant bioflavonoids *(p.89)*. This group of supplements may be helpful in preventing and, in some cases, helping to alleviate the symptoms of a disease.

NEW SUPPLEMENTS TO BENEFIT OUR HEALTH

Many of these supplements are relatively new to us, although scientists may have been aware of their potential benefits to human health for some time. In some cases, such as probiotics, results from clinical research suggest that they have a real benefit to our general health.

In other cases, scientific investigations are in early stages. While the research so far suggests a wide range of potential benefits, from reducing memory loss in old age to improving the chances of avoiding cataracts, more research needs to be conducted before we can be sure of all their actions in the body.

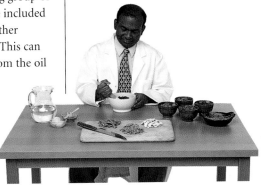

SUPPLEMENT PREPARATIONS

Not only are there a huge number of supplements now available on the market, they often come in a variety of forms: tablets to swallow or chew, capsules, liquids, powders, tinctures, infusions, or even gels.

Although you may feel overwhelmed by the choice of supplements on sale, the best advice is that where there is a choice, opt for the version you or your family find easiest to take.

TABLETS AND CAPSULES

Depending on the preparation, tablets and capsules contain not only the vitamin, mineral, or active ingredient of the herb, but also other substances known as "excipients." These are materials used in the process of tableting or encapsulating supplements, and can be grouped into four main classes:

FILLERS

As the name implies, fillers are used to increase the volume of material in a tablet or capsule; for example, vegetable oils. A vitamin supplement may contain only tiny quantities of the vitamin itself; if that were the only ingredient in a minuscule tablet, it would prove very difficult to handle. Fillers also provide an accurate potency of such minute quantities.

BINDERS

These substances cement together the nutrient component of tablets. Without binders, the tablet would crumble and fall apart.

DISINTEGRANTS

These substances help the tablet dissolve in the body's digestive tract, making it possible for the active ingredients to be absorbed effectively.

LUBRICANTS

Known as "flow agents" and "glidants," lubricants such as palm oil aid the removal of pressed tablets from machinery during the manufacturing process.

In addition, supplements may contain flavoring, sweeteners, coloring, and preservatives. Some companies, however, make a point of guaranteeing that their products are free from allergy-inducing excipients such as wheat, soy, gluten, grain, dairy produce, added sugars, preservatives, coloring,

CAPSULES AND TABLETS
Capsules and tablets make an easy-to-handle delivery system of active ingredients.

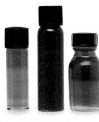

TINCTURES AND OILS
Supplements and herbal extracts can be delivered via tinctures, oils, syrups, and herbal teas, which may be easier to swallow.

yeast, or starch. It is also possible to find capsules that are made with vegetarian-based gels rather than animal-derived gelatin.

TIMED-RELEASE SUPPLEMENTS

Improved manufacturing processes have made it possible to produce timed-release tablets – also known as sustained release, and continuous release supplements. The active ingredients of the tablet are trickled gradually from the binding material rather than being released all at once.

This technology is particularly beneficial for water-soluble vitamins, which the body is unable to store. As the body's normal digestion proceeds, the tablet is eroded gradually and the nutrients are released over a six-hour period.

POWDERS AND OILS

Useful for those people who have difficulty in swallowing, powder and oil supplements can be mixed into water, juice, and, in some cases, food. Ground flax seeds form a powder consistency, for example, while cod liver oil and flavored evening primrose oil are available as oil in bottles and can be poured into a teaspoon to be swallowed directly.

CHELATED MINERALS

Minerals in supplements are bound, or chelated, to another substance – either inorganic, such as sulfates, carbonates, and phosphates – or organic, such as citrates, amino acids, or ascorbates. The chelation of minerals lets the mineral supplement pass through the stomach without causing upset, and prevents it from binding with other substances in the digestive tract that may alter its absorption.

The other, added substance can affect the absorption of a mineral; although research still continues, it is thought that minerals are best absorbed when chelated with amino acids.

POWDERS AND HERBS
In the case of ginger and peppermint, infusions or herbal drinks can be made either from the fresh herb or the dried root or leaves.

ABSORPTION HELPERS & HINDERERS

There are many factors that can affect the absorption of vitamins and minerals in the body, some of which enhance the effects and some which can actually inhibit the process.

Once a vitamin or mineral is consumed in food, drink, or via supplements, it must then be absorbed across the intestinal tract and into the bloodstream in order to work effectively in the body.

VITAMIN AND MINERAL SELF-HELPERS

To start with, vitamins and minerals themselves can have a positive absorption effect on one another. Taking vitamin C at the same time as vegetable-based foods that supply iron, for example, increases the absorption of this mineral. The same is true of combining vitamin D and calcium in the same meal. Taking the B vitamins as a complete group appears to enhance the absorption of each B vitamin, while vitamins A, C, and E appear to help the digestive tract absorb the mineral selenium.

OTHER NUTRITIONAL HELPERS

In the case of vitamin A and beta-carotene, the body finds both substances easier to absorb when they are eaten together with a little

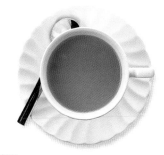

TEA
Tea contains health-promoting antioxidants, but drink it between meals as its tannins can reduce the absorption of iron from food.

oil or fat. Zinc absorption is also found to be improved if protein is included as part of the same meal.

VITAMIN AND MINERAL HINDERERS

In other situations, too much of one mineral, such as potassium, can impair the absorption of another mineral, like magnesium. In addition, other dietary factors can affect the absorption process:
● It is known that substances called "phytates," which are a type of fiber found in wholegrain cereal, can bind to a mineral such as zinc and pass it out of the body in the stools without being absorbed, while

tannin in tea binds to iron, making it unavailable for the body to absorb and use.

● Similarly, "oxalates" in rhubarb and spinach can bind themselves to calcium, rendering this mineral unavailable for use by the body.

● Drinking large amounts of cola, which has phosphorus-based additives, may affect calcium levels in the body. Large intakes of coffee may deplete levels of vitamin B1.

DRUGS

In some cases, the absorption of vitamins and minerals can also be adversely affected by prescription medications. In the case of vitamins D, E and K, the long-term use of a cholesterol-lowering drug known as cholestyramine has been proved to have such effects. Antacids taken to relieve indigestion can have a similar effect on vitamin A. The antidepressants imipramine and amitriptyline can lower the absorption of vitamin B2, while riboflavin and antibiotics, plus the drug l-dopamine, taken for Parkinson's disease, reduce the nutritional effectiveness of niacin.

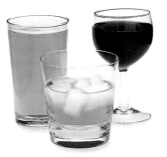

ALCOHOL
Regularly drinking more than the recommended amount of alcohol can reduce nutrient absorption and deplete body resources.

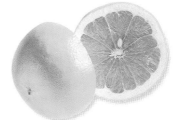

GRAPEFRUIT
Citrus fruits supply the body with vitamin C, which assists the absorption of iron in foods such as cereals, legumes, nuts, and seeds.

A BALANCING ACT

The key to good nutrition is getting the balance right and not to consume too much of one nutrient, which can unbalance the fine tuning of another. This list details certain nutrients with (i) nutrients that in adequate dietary intakes increase protection against deficiency, or (ii) substances that increase the risk of deficiency via excessive dietary intakes:

● **VITAMIN A**
(i) Vitamins C and E
(ii) Alcohol, iron, copper, manganese

● **VITAMIN D**
(i) Oil
(ii) Iron, manganese, copper

● **VITAMIN E**
(i) Vitamins C and selenium
(ii) Iron, manganese, copper

● **CALCIUM**
(i) Vitamin D, lactose, copper
(ii) Phytate, oxalate, phosphorus

● **PHOSPHORUS**
(i) Calcium, copper
(ii) Iron, aluminum

● **IRON**
(i) Vitamin C, folic acid, copper
(ii) Tannin, zinc, oxalate, phosphorus

● **ZINC**
(i) Protein
(ii) Iron, copper, calcium, phytate.

REASONS FOR TAKING SUPPLEMENTS

Some people get enough nutrients from their diet alone, but there will always be others who have low intakes of one or more nutrients, or who have special nutritional or medical needs for particular supplements at certain times.

BUSY, STRESSFUL LIFESTYLES

As the pace of adult life increases, diet may be one part of the jigsaw that gets neglected if you find yourself with little time to plan, shop, and eat a balanced diet. When this situation is exacerbated by additional nutritional needs resulting from stress, vitamin and mineral supplements may help repair the lack generated by a poor diet.

LIFESTAGES

Nutritional needs change throughout life. At certain lifestages, such as the period leading up to conception, during pregnancy, and while breastfeeding, for example, the body's need for certain vitamins, minerals, and other nutrients can significantly increase. In some cases, taking supplements may be the most practical and efficient – or only – way of making sure all nutritional requirements are met.

The same is true during other stages of life such as the teenage years, and in later life when the body's ability to absorb nutrients can decrease at a time when food intakes also decrease.

SMOKING

Certain lifestyles can increase the requirement of nutrients. Smoking, for example, soaks up the body's supplies of vitamin C, increasing the need for more of the vitamin in the diet. Since smokers notoriously have low intakes of vitamin C-rich foods, taking supplements before stopping the habit is a sensible step to take. Meanwhile, antioxidants such as selenium and vitamin E may help to protect the body against the lung damage

MOTHER AND CHILD
Before, during, and between pregnancies, it can be beneficial for women to top up their dietary intakes of vitamins, minerals, and essential fats with modest supplements. This will help them make sure their body stores do not become depleted.

that smoking and passive smoking cause. At the other end of the spectrum, people who undertake vigorous physical training may benefit from antioxidants to help neutralize the increased production of free radicals in the body, and to help maintain healthy blood, bones, and joints.

SPECIAL DIETS

Many people now opt for alterna-tive dietary patterns that may limit the variety of vitamins and minerals they can consume. For example, vegetarians and vegans who cut out foods from animal sources may find it hard to get their full complement of vitamins and minerals (and in adequate amounts) on a regular basis. For them, taking supplements may be a key to good health while still following their chosen plan.

Those people following reduced calorie plans and low-fat diets could also benefit from a multivitamin and mineral supplement to make sure all basic needs are being met.

"PREVENTATIVE EATING"

It is now becoming increasingly common for people to think about their health in terms of prevention, rather than waiting for a medical problem to arise. There is now some evidence to suggest that changing the way we eat and drink, and, in some cases, increasing intakes of certain nutrients to levels above those that are normally found in the diet, can reduce the possibility of disease in later life. Antioxidant nutrients

such as vitamins C and E, selenium, and bioflavonoids have attracted particular attention in this respect.

TREATING DISEASE

With the recent re-emergence of general interest in herbal medicine, many health practitioners and individuals are prepared to explore the herbal world for an answer to their health problems, rather than rely solely on prescription medicines. In such cases, it is vital that a qualified doctor makes a diagnosis prior to self-medication. The action of certain herbs may interact with prescription medicines, so advice should be sought, particularly if you already take drugs for a condition.

INSURANCE POLICY

Even those people who try to live healthily and eat a balanced diet may need a multivitamin and mineral supplement to make sure all their vitamin and mineral needs are met.

HEALTHY LIVING
People leading active lifestyles, and particularly those who take regular, strenuous exercise, can benefit from supplements to maintain their health and peak performance potential. Herbal and other supple–ments may also help to heal sport injuries.

Choosing & Using Supplements

Deciding on which supplement, and how much of it you should take, can be confusing. Having worked out why you wish to take a particular supplement, it is helpful to understand certain terms before making your decision.

In order to make sure you regulate the supplements you take, and don't hinder the absorption of other vitamins and minerals – or even cause unwanted side effects *(see also pp.14–15)* – official guidelines have been established to help you remain within safe limits of the supplement intake levels.

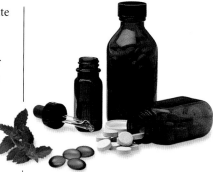

RDA

A figure known as RDA (Recommended Daily Allowances) indicates the basic – or minimum – amount of a particular substance you should be getting each day, either from the food you eat or from supplements. The RDA represents the amount of a vitamin or mineral needed by an average adult to maintain good health. The amount of a vitamin and mineral found in a supplement is often expressed as a percentage of the RDA. For example, a product supplying 60mg of vitamin C will provide 100 percent of the RDA for this nutrient. In the charts that follow, the RDAs are given for adults (female/male). The allowances for children, pregnant

SUPPLEMENT LABELS
Every pack of supplements lists an appropriate dose that will help maintain the health for the majority of people.

women, older people, and those on vegetarian diets may vary from these figures. Those people who fall into these categories should always check the relevant RDA in advance of taking supplements.

DRI

Over the next few years, a new standard is being phased in to replace RDA. "Dietary (Daily) Reference Intakes" represent an average of four different measures, which include the established RDA, the basic (minimum) requirement, the tolerable upper level, and the "average" intake.

OPTIMUM LEVELS

Some scientists believe that in order to achieve optimal mental and emotional balance, as well as optimal physical performance, the quantities of nutrients consumed should not be set at levels that simply maintain health and prevent deficiency disease.

Instead, they feel that intakes should be set at higher levels, which promote and maintain health at its optimum state. This, say optimum nutritionists, will improve an individual's mental clarity and concentration, increase his or her IQ, increase the ability to perform better physically, improve the quality of sleep, improve the body's resistance to infections, protect the immune system from disease, and extend a healthy lifespan.

SAFE UPPER LIMITS

Remember that everyone's requirements for supplements are different, and do not increase your intake sharply above the RDA or DRI without medical supervision.

OVERDOSING AND TOXICITY

It is never wise to exceed the recommended doses stated on the label of a supplement. While a small additional amount of a vitamin or mineral may sometimes be helpful, too much of any one supplement can cause health problems. Excessive intakes of vitamin A and many minerals such as selenium and zinc can be toxic and cause side effects. The same is true for some herbal remedies.

When combining supplements, be aware that you will need to add up the total intake of the nutrients they contain. You may unwittingly take too much vitamin D, for example, by consuming cod liver oil, a calcium and vitamin D supplement designed to improve bone condition, and a multivitamin and mineral supplement. If you are concerned about your total intake when combining supplements, ask the advice of a pharmacist or herbalist who will be able to make sure you stay within safe limits.

MEDICAL CHECKUPS

If you have a medical condition and are taking drugs, always consult a doctor before taking supplements. Equally, be sure to inform a doctor of any supplements you are already taking; supplements and drugs can adversely affect one another.

QUALITY PRODUCTS

When making your selection of supplements, try to choose brands that have been produced by established manufacturers with good reputations and quality-control procedures. Those companies who conduct clinical trials to prove the effectiveness of their products are particularly worth noting.

When purchasing herbal extracts, be sure to look for the words "standardized extract" on the label. This means that the manufacturer can guarantee that the product in question has a consistent potency and effectiveness.

YOUR VITAMIN & MINERAL INTAKE

It is not always easy to judge for yourself whether you are getting enough vitamins and mineral in your diet. Use this simple chart, and also the information on pp.22–23, to help you assess your intakes and supplement requirements.

	ANALYZING YOUR DIET	WHAT TO DO
1 A) Do you eat less than one serving of oily fish, yellow or green leafy vegetables, or liver per day? B) Do you have less than one serving of dairy products per day?	If either of your answers to these questions were "yes," you may not be getting enough Vitamin A. If you answered "yes" to both, the risk of vitamin A deficiency is greater.	Try to eat more dairy products, liver, and sources of beta-carotene such as dark green leafy vegetables, carrots, or tomatoes, which the body can convert into vitamin A.
2 A) Do you eat less than one serving of starchy foods per day, namely bread, legumes, rice, pasta, or cereals? B) Do you have less than two servings of meat, eggs, or liver per day? C) Do you often eat out for your main meals, or eat on the run?	If any of your answers to this question were "yes," you may not be getting enough B-complex vitamins. If you answered "yes" to two or more of the questions, the risk of vitamin B deficiency is greater.	Try to eat more wholegrain products, yeast extract, fortified breakfast cereals, variety meats, legumes, and dairy products. Restaurant food may be low in B vitamins, which are destroyed by cooking and in food that is kept warm.
3 A) Do you have less than two or three servings of fruit per day? B) Do you smoke? C) Are you consuming less than two or three servings of raw or slightly cooked vegetables per day? D) Do you often eat out for your main meals, or eat on the run?	If you answered "yes" to any part of question 3, you may not be getting enough vitamin C. There is a greater risk of vitamin C deficiency if you answered "yes" to more than two of these questions.	Try to eat more fruit (particularly citrus fruit), juices, tomatoes, and vegetables. Try to avoid food that has been overcooked or prepared a long time in advance, because their vitamin C content is likely to be low.

	ANALYZING YOUR DIET	**WHAT TO DO**
A) Do you have less than one serving of oily fish, breakfast cereal, or eggs per day? **B)** Do you avoid using fats such as butter? **C)** Do you rarely go out in the sunlight or expose little skin when outside?	Answering "yes" to a, b, or c could mean that you may not be getting enough vitamin D. If more than one of your answers was "yes," the risk of vitamin deficiency is greater.	An easy way of boosting your vitamin D intake is to expose your skin to sunlight. If this is not possible, you should include eggs, oily fish, and butter in your diet.
A) Do you regularly have less than one serving of red meat, dried fruit, eggs, lentils, nuts, or liver per day? **B)** Do you eat fewer than two slices of bread per day? **C)** Do you consume fewer than three servings of fruit and vegetables per day?	You may not be getting enough iron if you answered "yes" to any of these questions. Again, if you answered "yes" to more than one, your risk of iron deficiency is higher.	Eating more dried fruit, eggs, nuts, lentils, and small servings of red meat and liver will increase your levels of iron. The absorption of iron is increased by vitamin C, so it is important to eat plenty of fruit and vegetables.
A) Do you eat less than two servings of dairy produce or oily fish per day? **B)** Do you rarely eat green leafy vegetables or bread? **C)** Did you answer "yes" to more than one question in number 5?	If you answered "yes" to any part of question 6, you may not be getting enough calcium. Answering "yes" to more than one will increase the risk of calcium deficiency.	Try to eat more low-fat dairy products (e.g. milk, yogurt, cheese), eggs, leafy vegetables, canned pilchards, and sardines. Vegans and those who choose not to eat dairy produce should eat plenty of nuts, legumes, dried fruit, and cereals.
A) Do you seldom eat grains, cereal, meat, or liver? **B)** Do you eat a lot of fiber e.g., you always choose wholewheat bread, brown rice, wholewheat pasta, and wholewheat breakfast cereals?	If either of your answers for question 7 were "yes," you may not be getting enough zinc.	Eating more nuts, peas, beans, small portions of meat, liver, seafood – especially crab meat – and oysters will boost your levels of zinc.

PART ONE

CREATING A PERSONAL PROGRAM

Everyone's nutritional needs are different and are dependent on many factors: stress, how well you eat, whether you drink too much alcohol, have a particular health problem, or even whether you get a regular dose of sunshine.

Even if you are generally healthy and eat a balanced diet most of the time, supplementing your diet with a multivitamin and mineral tablet or capsule that supplies 100 percent of the recommended daily allowance can still be appropriate.

These extra benefits can help you make sure that any nutritional shortfalls, which may still occur from time to time, are covered, and can also raise intakes of nutrients from minimum or satisfactory levels to doses that may actually help to optimize your health.

FOOD DIARY

No one food can make for a healthy diet. In short, you need to eat a variety of foods from different groups or sources. Balancing your diet is not as hard as it may first appear. Selecting foods in the following proportions helps achieve a good balance for everyone over the age of five years (the number of servings chosen depends on size, sex, and activity levels):

◆ **GRAINS**
Bread, cereal, pasta, rice: 6–11 servings per day.

◆ **VEGETABLES**
Whole vegetables, vegetable dishes and soup: 3–5 servings per day.

◆ **FRUITS**
Whole fruits, fruit juice, fruit dishes such as fruit salad: 2–4 servings per day.

◆ **MILK FOODS**
Milk, yogurt, cheese, calcium-enriched soy products: 2–3 servings per day.

◆ **MEAT GROUP**
Meat, poultry, fish, beans, tofu, eggs, nuts, seeds: 2 servings per day.

Jot down everything you eat and drink over one week. At the end of this time, look back and count the number of servings of food you

SUPPLEMENTS
Sometimes it is useful to boost your dietary vitamin intake with supplements.

had from each food group. If you are short of, or having too much of, a particular group, try to correct the imbalance in your diet and check the list below for the nutrients you could be missing out on.

GRAINS:
B vitamins, vitamin E, zinc, selenium, calcium, iron, chromium, manganese, copper, fiber.

VEGETABLES:
Vitamin C, betacarotene and vitamin A, B vitamins, vitamin E, vitamin K, potassium, calcium, magnesium, iron, copper, molybdenum, chromium, bioflavonoids, carotenes, fiber.

FRUIT:
Vitamin C, potassium, betacarotene, other carotenes, bioflavonoids.

DAIRY FOODS:
Vitamin A, B vitamins, vitamin D, calcium, phosphorus, magnesium.

MEAT GROUP:
Vitamin D, B vitamins, iron, zinc, selenium, copper.

PRECAUTIONS

If you are unsure about which supplements are appropriate for your needs, seek professional help from a dietician, nutritionist, your own doctor, or a pharmacist or doctor with a specialized understanding of supplements. If you have medical problems or take prescription drugs, check with your doctor before taking supplements.

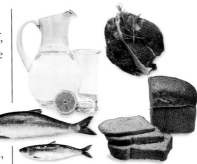

MINERALS
The small amounts of minerals needed by the body can be obtained from foods.

PERSONAL PREFERENCES

Having decided upon which supplements you wish to take, the key to getting any benefit is to take them on a regular basis and to feel comfortable with your program. Ask yourself these questions and decide which form of supplement best suits you, and when to take it:

• **Do you have a regular routine?**
Make sure your supplements are part of any daily routine you have.

• **Do supplements make you queasy?**
Take the supplements before a meal.

• **Do tablets get stuck in your throat?**
Buy powdered or chewable tablets, liquid, or lozenges. Or buy 500mg rather than 1000mg (1g) versions.

• **Do you take several supplements?**
Put your day's supplements together in a container.

VITAMINS
A healthy diet provides vitamins that are crucial for maintaining good health.

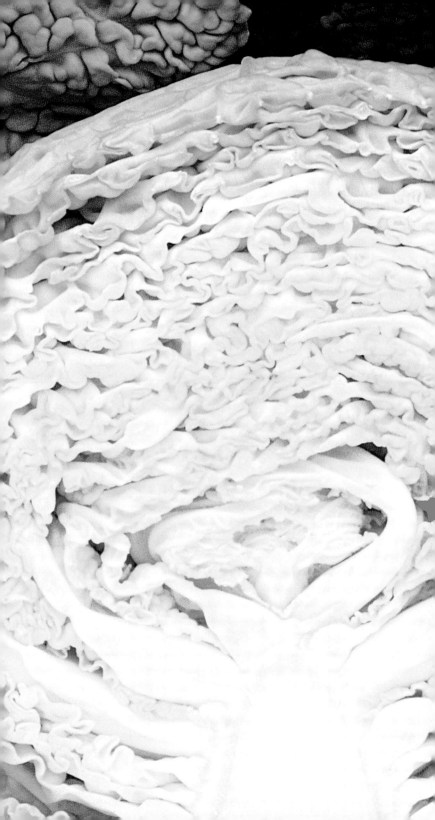

Guide to Vitamins

Vitamins are organic substances, crucial for human health; a lack of any vitamin in the body leads to a corresponding deficiency disease. Optimizing vitamin intakes may help to maintain good health and slow down the aging process.

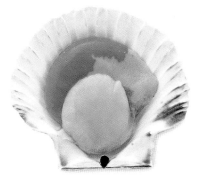

VITAMIN A/RETINOL

Promotes healthy skin and good night vision

Strengthens immune system ◆ Can help treat acne

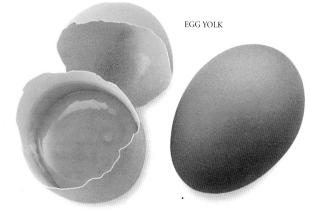

EGG YOLK

CHEMICAL NAMES

- RETINOL
- RETINOL PALMITATE
- RETINOL ACETATE

PREPARATIONS

- CAPSULES
- TABLETS
- LIQUID
- COD LIVER OIL

RDA FOR ADULTS

- 800/1000MCG

HOW IT WORKS

Vitamin A is needed by the body for the production of rhodpsin, a pigment that enables us to see in the dark. It is also crucial for keeping the linings of the mouth and lungs moist, the adequate growth of body tissues, and maintaining the development of strong bones, a balanced reproductive system, and healthy skin. It also plays a role in the body's immune response, helping fight bacterial, viral, and parasitic infections.

ABSORPTION HELPERS

Vitamin A is best absorbed together with a little oil or fat in the diet.

ABSORPTION INHIBITORS

Long-term use of the drug cholestyramine, which is prescribed for the treatment of high cholesterol, can alter the natural balance of vitamin A in the body. Antacids required for indigestion may also reduce the body's vitamin A stores, and a lack of the mineral zinc in the diet may lower blood levels.

TOP SOURCES OF VITAMIN A mcg/4oz. of food

CALVES' LIVER
29,730mcg/4oz.

BUTTER
815mcg/4oz.

MARGARINE
780mcg/4oz.

EGG YOLK
535mcg/4oz.

CREAM CHEESE
385mcg/4oz.

TAKING VITAMIN A SUPPLEMENTS

The RDA (800/1000mcg) for vitamin A is equivalent to 3 grams of broiled calves' liver, or eight eggs. The body can also make vitamin A from beta-carotene, the bright pigment in vegetables and fruit *(see p.91)*. Vitamin A supplements are usually oil based and derived from fish oils. Vitamin A is also present in cod liver oil.

PRECAUTIONS

Vitamin A is stored in the body's fat cells, so excess intakes build up over time and can become toxic. Doses of 300mg in adults and 100mg in children are harmful, causing hair loss, vomiting, headaches, bone damage, double vision, and liver damage. Regular intakes should not exceed 9,000mcg in men and 7,500mcg in women; the best advice is to not exceed 100 percent of the RDA. Avoid combining vitamin A sources – such as multivitamins plus cod liver oil – which together may contribute to excess intakes. Supplements should be avoided by pregnant women; intakes of 3,300mcg a day can cause birth defects in the developing fetus.

THERAPEUTIC USES

● **PSORIASIS AND ACNE**
Psoriasis and acne may improve from high doses of vitamin A by helping to change the way the skin's surface is formed. This must be done under a doctor's supervision.

● **CANCER**
The action of substances that trigger cancerous changes to cells in the body may be dampened down if vitamin A is in good supply. If vitamin A stores are low, supplements may help to prevent the risk of developing cancer.

● **RESPIRATORY PROBLEMS**
Vitamin A supplements may reduce the number of respiratory illnesses in children who regularly suffer this condition.

● **GLAUCOMA**
It is possible that vitamin A supplements may be beneficial to those with glaucoma if the vitamin is lacking in the diet.

● **MEASLES**
A course of supplements may dramatically reduce the risk of measles in children whose diets are poor in vitamin A.

WHY TAKE THIS SUPPLEMENT?

Anyone on a long-term low-fat diet, or with poor absorption (such as people with cystic fibrosis), or taking cholestyramine may benefit from this supplement. Specialist skin doctors may prescribe a course of vitamin A supplements, and people with the following symptoms may have vitamin A deficiency:

❍ INCREASED SUSCEPTIBILITY TO INFECTIONS
❍ INABILITY TO ADJUST EYESIGHT TO SEE IN THE DARK
❍ POOR GROWTH IN CHILDHOOD
❍ DRY, SCALY SKIN
❍ DISLIKE OF LIGHT
❍ DULL, DRY EYES
❍ GINGIVITIS
❍ FOLLICULAR HYPERKERATOSIS (BUMPS ON HAIR FOLICLES ON SKIN'S SURFACE)
❍ TOOTH ENAMEL DEVELOPS POORLY IN CHILDREN

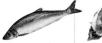

HERRING
45mcg/4oz.

OYSTERS
75mcg/4oz.

ANCHOVIES
57mcg/4oz.

WHOLE MILK
52mcg/4oz.

MACKEREL
45mcg/4oz.

VITAMIN B1/THIAMIN

Improves memory ◆ Needed for
nerve health ◆ Helps reduce sugar cravings

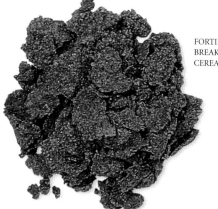

FORTIFIED
BREAKFAST
CEREAL

CHEMICAL NAMES

• THIAMIN

PREPARATIONS

• CAPSULES
• TABLETS

RDA FOR ADULTS

• 1.1/1.5MG

HOW IT WORKS

Vitamin B1, also known as thiamin, is essential for the transmission of certain types of nerve signals between the brain and the spinal cord. It is also crucial for the workings of particular types of enzymes that make energy available in the body. Body stores are relatively small so regular intakes are vital.

ABSORPTION HELPERS

Vitamin C and citric acid, found in oranges and other citrus fruits, may help to prevent thiamin destruction, while B vitamins tend to work together to enhance one another's absorption.

ABSORPTION INHIBITORS

Long-term intakes of antacids reduce B1 levels in the body, as do high intakes of alcohol. Caffeic acids in coffee, tannic acids in tea, and sulfur dioxide used in the drying of fruit adversely affects vitamin B1 absorption and destroy thiamin. Eating sushi regularly may

TOP SOURCES OF VITAMIN B1 mg/4oz. of food

YEAST
EXTRACT
4.25mg/4oz.

PEAS
0.89mg/4oz.

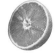

ORANGES
0.70mg/4oz.

FORTIFIED
CORNFLAKES
0.65mg/4oz.

BOILED
POTATOES
0.59mg/4oz.

reduce absorption since raw fish contains thiamin-breaking enzymes.

TAKING THIAMIN SUPPLEMENTS

The adult RDA for thiamin (1.1/1.5mg a day) is equivalent to one bowl of fortified breakfast cereal or a serving of pork. Large single doses of thiamin are poorly absorbed by the body, so it is best to have 100 percent of the RDA on a regular basis. No long- or short-term effects have been established in adults taking up to 100mg supplements a day. Optimum nutritionists recommend 3.5–9.2mg per day to maintain health, and 25–100mg a day for therapeutic use.

COMBINING SUPPLEMENTS

Taking vitamin B1 supplements together with vitamins B2 and B6 appears to help B1 to work more effectively in the body.

PRECAUTIONS

Intakes greater than 25mg per pound of bodyweight, or 3g per day have been shown to be toxic. Such levels have led to symptoms such as a rapid pulse, inability to sleep, general weakness, headaches, and irritability. Too much thiamin may lead to the loss of other B vitamins from the body.

THERAPEUTIC USES

● IMPROVED MEMORY

Thiamin is necessary for the glucose in the blood to produce a substance called acetylcholine, which transmits messages between nerves and is crucial for the memory and for concentration levels. It has been suggested that eating a breakfast that includes both carbohydrate, which increases blood glucose levels, and thiamin, which facilitates acetylcholine production, may lead to improved memory functioning in the morning ahead.

● DECREASED SUGAR CRAVINGS

A mild deficiency of thiamin may lead to sugar cravings, which could be improved through a modest intake of the supplement.

● ALZHEIMER'S DISEASE

New studies have shown that thiamin supplements might be helpful for preventing and slowing Alzheimer's disease – essentially a disease of aging – which is characterized by forgetfulness.

● MULTIPLE SCLEROSIS

Doctors may prescribe thiamin supplements to treat a range of disorders of the nervous system, such as the disease multiple sclerosis, Bell's palsy, and neuritis.

WHY TAKE THIS SUPPLEMENT?

Full-blown thiamin deficiency, known as beriberi, is unusual in western countries. Alcoholism is a main cause of thiamin deficiency, but those with a stressful lifestyle, physically active people, and those over 55 may benefit from taking supplements. B1 deficiency may trigger:

○ TIREDNESS
○ DEPRESSION
○ POOR MEMORY
○ HEADACHES
○ NAUSEA
○ TINGLING HANDS

WHOLEWHEAT PASTA
0.43mg/4oz.

WHOLEWHEAT BREAD
0.37mg/4oz.

EGG YOLK
0.30mg/4oz.

WHITE BREAD
0.21mg/4oz.

PORK CHOP
0.48mg/4oz.

VITAMIN B2/RIBOFLAVIN

Improves energy levels ✦ Maintains healthy skin

Keeps nails and hair healthy ✦ May alleviate pregnancy cramps

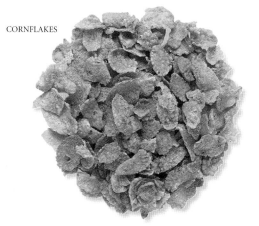

CORNFLAKES

CHEMICAL NAMES

- RIBOFLAVIN

PREPARATIONS

- TABLETS
- CAPSULES

RDA FOR ADULTS

- 1.3/1.8MG

HOW IT WORKS

Riboflavin is needed by the body to form two substances that are vital for turning the calories from protein, fat, and carbohydrate in food into a form that cells can use efficiently: FAD – which stands for flavin adenine dinucleotide; and FMN – which stands for flavin mononucleotide. (A lack of riboflavin in the body reduces energy levels.) Riboflavin is also needed for the formation of hair, skin, and nails.

ABSORPTION HELPERS

Riboflavin is best absorbed in the presence of other B vitamins and the mineral selenium, found in Brazil nuts, red meat, and wholegrain cereals.

ABSORPTION INHIBITORS

High intakes of alcohol, antidepressant drugs such as imipramine and amitriptyline, the drug adfiamycin used in chemotherapy, and the antimalarial drug quinacrine can all reduce absorption of riboflavin.

TOP SOURCES OF VITAMIN B2 mg/4oz. of food

   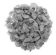

YEAST EXTRACT	LAMB'S LIVER	PORK KIDNEY	FORTIFIED CORNFLAKES	CHEDDAR CHEESE
11.0mg/4oz.	4.4mg/4oz.	2.1mg/4oz.	1.3mg/4oz.	0.4mg/4oz.

Too much iron, zinc, copper, or manganese has a similar effect. Smoking and the contraceptive pill may also deplete levels in the body, while the exposure of foods to sunlight can destroy this vitamin before being consumed.

TAKING RIBOFLAVIN SUPPLEMENTS

The RDA (1.3/1.8mg) can be obtained from eating two large bowls of fortified cereal with skimmed milk. 200mg of riboflavin a day is set as a safe upper limit. Optimum nutritionists believe that intakes of 1.8–2.5mg a day are appropriate, and 25–100mg daily for therapeutic uses are suggested.

COMBINING SUPPLEMENTS

Riboflavin is best taken with food as a vitamin B-complex supplement.

PRECAUTIONS

People with, or who are prone to, cataracts should not take more than 10mg daily because the combination of light, oxygen, and riboflavin increases the risk of cataract development. High doses may increase the risk of magnesium

deficiency. Since there are no benefits to taking mega doses, intakes should not exceed 200mg a day.

THERAPEUTIC USES

● ANEMIA
Research indicates that riboflavin, used in conjunction with iron, enhances iron therapy and improves anemia.

● CANDIDIASIS
Sufferers with low levels of riboflavin may benefit from supplementation.

● CARPAL TUNNEL SYNDROME
Riboflavin is needed with vitamin B6 to treat Carpal Tunnel Syndrome. A lack of riboflavin can stop vitamin B6 from working, a problem that can be resolved by taking riboflavin supplements.

● CATARACTS
While excess riboflavin increases the risk of cataracts, too little may also be a problem. Improvements may occur by taking modest supplements over a period of nine months.

● PREGNANCY CRAMPS
Pain relief may occur if 10mg of riboflavin supplements are taken daily.

WHY TAKE THIS SUPPLEMENT?

The amount of riboflavin lost in the urine tends to increase in people who are stressed or have diabetes. They may therefore need more of this vitamin. Women taking the oral contraceptive pill may experience similar effects, while vegans (who consume no animal foods), the elderly, and those who are dieting may have poor intakes. Riboflavin depletion is also common in pregnant women. Poor intakes can also lead to the following symptoms:
- TREMBLING
- DIZZINESS
- POOR CONCENTRATION
- WEAKNESS
- BLOODSHOT, TIRED, RED, AND GRITTY EYES
- INFLAMED TONGUE AND LIPS
- ECZEMALIKE SKIN RASH
- SPLIT NAILS
- DULL OR OILY HAIR
- HAIR LOSS
- CATARACTS

EGGS
0.35mg/4oz.

BEEF
0.33mg/4oz.

YOGURT
0.27mg/4oz.

CHICKEN
0.19mg/4oz.

WHOLE MILK
0.17mg/4oz.

VITAMIN B3/NIACIN

Lowers high cholesterol ◆ May help people with high

alcoholic intakes ◆ Can help improve acne rosacea

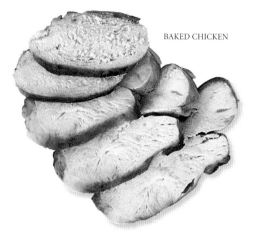

BAKED CHICKEN

CHEMICAL NAMES

- NIACIN
- NICOTINIC ACID
- NICOTINAMIDE

PREPARATIONS

- TABLETS
- CAPSULES
- POWDER

RDA FOR ADULTS

- 15/20MG

HOW IT WORKS

Niacin is needed by the body for the production of two enzymes known as NAD and NADP, which help energy to be released from digested food. Needs for niacin increase with greater physical activity. This vitamin can also be produced in the body from a protein "building block" called tryptophan. Niacin is involved in the normal growth of skin, the formation of healthy nerves, and maintaining a good digestive system.

ABSORPTION HELPERS

Good dietary intakes of tryptophan (which is found in dairy foods, meat, and eggs) can help to improve levels of niacin, while other B vitamins and the mineral chromium can improve its absorption. Niacin is best taken as a B-complex supplement with food.

ABSORPTION INHIBITORS

Antibiotics used to treat bacterial infections, the drug l-dopamine for people with Parkinson's

TOP SOURCES OF VITAMIN B3 mg/4oz. of food

CHICKEN	PORK	BEEF	WHEATGERM	TURKEY
12.8mg/4oz.	11.0mg/4oz.	10.2mg/4oz.	9.8mg/4oz.	8.5mg/4oz.

disease, alcohol, the contraceptive pill, tea, and coffee may all reduce levels of niacin in the body.

TAKING NIACIN SUPPLEMENTS

The adult RDA for niacin (15/20mg) is equivalent to one portion of mixed nuts, baked chicken, and a serving of cornflakes. Niacin supplements are available as nicotinic acid and nicotinamide. The safe upper intake for nicotinamide is 1500mg in the short term and 450mg for the long term, while nicotinic acid is 500mg in the short term and 150mg for the long term. Optimum nutritionists set daily recommended intakes of nicotinic acid at 25–30mg a day and therapeutic levels of 50–150mg a day.

PRECAUTIONS

Very high intakes of 3–6g of nicotinic acid damage the liver, while intakes of more than 150mg a day of nicotinic acid may cause temporary flushing of the skin in some people. If taken as nicotinamide, this effect does not occur, although large intakes of nicotinamide can cause sedation. Those who suffer from gout should avoid supplements.

THERAPEUTIC USES

● ACNE ROSACEA

A skin condition causing flushing on the face, particularly in menopausal women, acne rosacea is caused by the expansion of tiny blood vessels under the skin, which leads to an "overgrowth" of oil-producing glands, causing acnelike spots. Daily supplementation may improve the condition.

● REDUCTION IN ALCOHOLIC CRAVINGS

Cravings for alcohol have been shown to be lowered with 500-1000mg niacin capsules, taken for three to four weeks.

● ALLERGIC REACTIONS

Niacin appears to inhibit the release of histamine and may also lead to a rapid improvement in hay fever symptoms.

● HEART DISEASE

Low doses of niacin may increase the protective form of cholesterol known as "HDL" cholesterol and help reduce the buildup of sticky, blocking plaques on the artery walls. Doses of niacin must only be taken under guidance of a doctor because of any potential side effects, and must not be used by people with diabetes who also have symptoms of heart disease.

● ASTHMA

Asthma may be improved with daily supplements of 100–200mg of niacin.

WHY TAKE THIS SUPPLEMENT?

Older people with a poor diet and an aging digestive system may benefit from this supplement, while those leading busy and stressful lives and the physically active also have increased needs. Deficiency of niacin leads to the disease pellagra; the following symptoms might also indicate the need for extra niacin:

○ LOSS OF APPETITE
○ HEADACHES
○ NAUSEA
○ MOUTH ULCERS
○ DRY SKIN
○ DIFFICULTY IN SLEEPING
○ POOR MEMORY
○ IRRITABILITY
○ SENSITIVITY TO STRONG LIGHT
○ INFLAMED GUMS
○ REDDENED TONGUE

CHEDDAR CHEESE
0.4mg/4oz.

WHOLEWHEAT BREAD
5.9mg/4oz.

COD
5.7mg/4oz.

LAMB CHOPS
4.8mg/4oz.

EGGS
3.8mg/4oz.

VITAMIN B5 / PANTOTHENIC ACID

May speed up the healing of wounds ✦ May help to alleviate the symptoms of rheumatoid arthritis

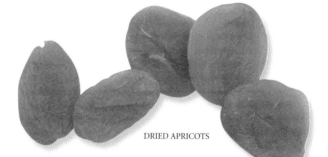

DRIED APRICOTS

CHEMICAL NAMES

- PANTOTHENIC ACID
- PANTETHINE
- CALCIUM PANTOTHENATE

PREPARATIONS

- TABLETS
- CAPSULES
- LIQUID

RDA FOR ADULTS

- 6MG

HOW IT WORKS

Pantothenic acid helps provide the body with a constant supply of energy to every cell. It does so by assisting in the creation of a molecule that converts the fat and sugar in food into a form that cells can use. It also helps support normal growth and assists the body in fighting infection by producing antibodies. Pantothenic acid is involved in the synthesis of antistress hormones in the adrenal glands, so helping to keep us calm.

ABSORPTION HELPERS

Pantothenic acid is best absorbed when taken with other B vitamins as a B-complex supplement taken with food. Folic acid and biotin in particular improve its absorption.

ABSORPTION INHIBITORS

Stress, too much alcohol, and large quantities of tea and coffee may all reduce the absorption of pantothenic acid, while heat and food processing reduces the amount found in foods.

TOP SOURCES OF VITAMIN B5 mg/4oz. of food

CALVES' LIVER	PLAIN PEANUTS	TAHINI PASTE	SESAME SEEDS	PECANS
8.4mg/4oz.	2.66mg/4oz.	2.17mg/4oz.	2.14mg/4oz.	1.71mg/4oz.

TAKING PANTOTHENIC ACID SUPPLEMENTS

The safe upper limit for both short- and long-term usage of pantothenic acid is 1,000mg. Optimum nutritionists advise intakes of 25mg a day for adults and a therapeutic intake of 50–300mg daily.

PRECAUTIONS

Excessively high intakes of 10,000mg (10g) have been known to cause diarrhea and other intestinal disturbances, while intakes of 100mg daily may increase the risk of niacin being excreted in the urine.

THERAPEUTIC USES

● **ALLERGIC REACTIONS**
Patients with an allergic inflammation of the nasal passages – causing a runny, itchy nose – may find almost instant relief after taking 250mg pantothenic acid. Studies have shown this is due to its antihistamine effect in the body.

● **CONSTIPATION**
Pantothenic acid helps to stimulate the contractions of the bowel, which leads to defecation. Supplements relieve constipation and provide an alternative to prescribed drugs for pregnant women, children, and the elderly.

● **FATIGUE**
Supplementing a poor diet with 10mg of pantothenic acid daily reduces fatigue and improves low moods and insomnia. It is also useful for treating post-surgical tiredness.

● **HEALING**
Taken with vitamin C, pantothenic acid appears to help strengthen the skin, promote the healing of recent cuts, and improve the durability of scars. It may also speed up healing following surgery.

● **RESPIRATORY INFECTIONS**
A lack of pantothenic acid in the diet may increase the risk of infections in the ear, nose, and throat. Supplements will correct any deficiency.

● **RHEUMATOID ARTHRITIS**
Levels of pantothenic acid may be low in people who have rheumatoid arthritis. Research indicates that these sufferers may benefit from taking 2g of calcium pantothenate on a daily basis. Increase intakes gradually by 500mg on the advice of a doctor.

WHY TAKE THIS SUPPLEMENT?

Pantothenic acid is widely available from a range of foods. However, those people who consume large amounts of alcohol, or who suffer from prolonged stress, or who have recently undergone surgery may all benefit from taking pantothenic acid supplements. The following symptoms may also indicate the need for extra levels of pantothenic acid in the body:

○ POOR MUSCLE COORDINATION AND TREMORS
○ MUSCLE CRAMPS
○ NUMBNESS
○ TINGLING
○ PAINFUL, BURNING FEET AND TENDER HEELS
○ DEPRESSION
○ EXHAUSTION AND FATIGUE
○ WEAKNESS
○ ANXIETY
○ NIGHTTIME TEETH GRINDING
○ HEADACHES
○ LOSS OF APPETITE

WALNUTS
1.6mg/4oz.

AVOCADO
1.1mg/4oz.

APPLES
0.7mg/4oz.

DRIED APRICOTS
0.7mg/4oz.

DRIED FIGS
0.51mg/4oz.

VITAMIN B6/PYRIDOXINE

Helps ease premenstrual syndrome ◆ Improves carpal tunnel syndrome ◆ Improves low moods and fatigue

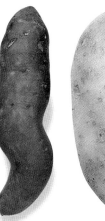

SWEET POTATO

WHITE POTATO

CHEMICAL NAMES

- PYRIDOXINE
- PYRIDOXAL-5-PHOSPHATE (P-5-P)
- PYRIDOXINE HYDROCHLORIDE

PREPARATIONS

- TABLETS
- CAPSULES
- LIQUID

RDA FOR ADULTS

- 1.5/2MG

HOW IT WORKS

Vitamin B6 is used by the body in its metabolism of protein to make and repair muscle and other tissues, and in the production of enzymes. It also appears to play a role in the balancing of sex hormones, which is why it is popular with women suffering premenstrual symptoms. Vitamin B6 is needed for healthy skin, for keeping the nervous system in good working order, and for the formation of antibodies, which fight infection. The vitamin also assists in the making of the red oxygen carrying blood pigment, called hemoglobin.

ABSORPTION HELPERS

Other B vitamins and the minerals magnesium and zinc help its absorption.

ABSORPTION INHIBITORS

Penicillin can bind to vitamin B6, so reducing its absorption. Alcohol, the contraceptive pill, and smoking may also reduce its levels in the body.

TOP SOURCES OF VITAMIN B6 mg/4oz. of food

WHEATGERM	WHEATBRAN	OX LIVER	COD	TURKEY
3.3mg/4oz.	1.38mg/4oz.	0.83mg/4oz.	0.38mg/4oz.	0.32mg/4oz.

TAKING SUPPLEMENTS

The adult RDA of vitamin B6 (1.5/2mg) can easily be obtained by eating a meal of salmon with a baked potato. It is also safe, however, to take up to 100mg a day on a long-term basis. This might be considered by women attempting to damp down symptoms of pre-menstrual syndrome and also by those women taking the combined contraceptive pill. Optimum nutritionists believe that levels of 2–5mg daily for children and 50–250mg a day for adults are appropriate. Pyridoxine is the best form in which to take B6, although pyridoxal-5-phosphate is also accept-able if it is enterically coated (to avoid being digested in the stomach).

PRECAUTIONS

The body only absorbs around 100mg of vitamin B6 at a time. Rare reports of toxicity at intakes of 200mg a day have occurred, which can lead to neuritis, a painful inflammation of the nerves. Vitamin B6 can also interfere with the drug levadopa, taken by people with Parkinson's disease.

THERAPEUTIC USES

● **PREMENSTRUAL SYNDROME (PMS)**
Many women claim that vitamin B6 can reduce their symptoms of pre-menstrual tension – such as mood swings and depression. While not yet conclusively proven with scientific research, opti-mum intakes of 50–250mg a day may be beneficial.

● **CARPAL TUNNEL SYNDROME (CPS)**
The numbness, tingling, and pain experienced in the hands of those with carpal tunnel syndrome may be improved with vitamin B6 supplements.

● **LOW MOODS**
Vitamin B6 is needed for the production of the feel-good nerve transmitter, called serotonin, in the brain. People who suffer from depression have been found to have lower blood levels of vitamin B6, so supplementation may be beneficial.

● **FATIGUE**
A supplement supplying the B-complex vitamins, including vitamin B6, may help to improve symptoms of tiredness and fatigue.

WHY TAKE THIS SUPPLEMENT?

Vitamin B6 is excreted in the urine just eight hours after entering the body, so regular intakes are beneficial. Deficiency is rare in developed countries, although women on the combined contra-ceptive pill, people over 55 in whom intestinal absorption may be reduced, vegetarians, vegans, people eating a high protein diet, and those consuming large amounts of alcohol may benefit. The following symptoms may also indicate a need for supplements:

○ PREMENSTRUAL SYMPTOMS
○ GENERAL IRRITABILITY
○ STRESS
○ NERVOUSNESS
○ LOW MOODS
○ LACK OF ENERGY
○ FLAKY, DRY SKIN
○ ANEMIA
○ DRY, CRACKED LIPS
○ INFLAMED TONGUE
○ BURNING SENSATION OF THE SKIN
○ INFLAMED EYELIDS

BEEF
0.30mg/4oz.

BANANA
0.29mg/4oz.

BRUSSELS SPROUTS
0.19mg/4oz.

CABBAGE
0.17mg/4oz.

MANGO
0.13mg/4oz.

B12/COBALAMIN

Prevents anemia ● Promotes growth

Maintains healthy nervous system ● Relieves irritability

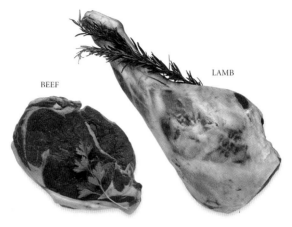

BEEF

LAMB

CHEMICAL NAMES

• COBALAMIN

PREPARATIONS

• TABLETS
• CAPSULES

RDA FOR ADULTS

• 2MCG

HOW IT WORKS

Vitamin B12 is crucial for the recycling of certain key enzymes in the body, which help to maintain the health of nerves and other cells. It is needed to create the "myelin sheath," a covering around nerves that allows for the quick transmission of nerve impulses. B12 is also needed for growth when we are young, is involved in controlling the appetite, and is necessary for the production of healthy red blood cells.

ABSORPTION HELPERS

The mineral calcium and other B vitamins, as well as vitamins A, C, and E, all work together to improve B12 absorption in the body.

ABSORPTION INHIBITORS

Certain drugs used to treat non-insulin dependent diabetics, Cholestyramine (used to treat high cholesterol), and the oral contraceptive pill all reduce B12 absorption. Sleeping pills and alcohol have a similar effect.

TOP TEN NATURAL SOURCES mcg/4oz.

LAMB'S LIVER	LIVER PATE	PORK	DUCK	PHEASANT
81mcg/4oz.	7.2mcg/4oz.	2mcg/4oz.	3mcg/4oz.	2.5mcg/4oz.

TAKING B12 SUPPLEMENTS

The adult RDA for vitamin B12 (2mcg) a day is equivalent to one 2oz. serving of beef. Intakes of vitamin B12 can be sustained by regularly eating foods such as meat, poultry, fish, eggs, dairy foods, fortified breakfast cereals, and also fortified yeast extract.

Cyanocobalamin is the best form of vitamin B12 supplement to take. While only 1mcg is needed daily in order to prevent deficiency of B12 in the body, the optimum amount suggested for this vitamin is 2.5–25mcg daily for children and 5–10mcg for adults.

COMBINING SUPPLEMENTS

Vitamin B12 works well in conjunction with folic acid and is best taken as a B-complex supplement with food.

PRECAUTIONS

No side effects of vitamin B12 are known at present. The safe upper level for the vitamin has been established at 3,000mcg a day; no long- or short-term toxicity problems have yet been established for this amount.

THERAPEUTIC USES

● IMPROVED MOOD

Vitamin B12 appears to be indirectly important in the production of brain transmitters – such as the "feel good" substances serotonin and dopamine. As these chemicals are able to control our moods, sleep patterns, and other psychological functions, B12 supplements may improve low moods.

● FATIGUE

Doctors now use vitamin B12 supplements and injections for a wide range of problems that affect energy levels.

● DIABETES

The nerve damage experienced by people who have diabetes is similar to the deficiency symptoms of B12. Some researchers believe that a disturbance in the B12 metabolism in diabetics might increase nerve damage, so supplements may be appropriate.

● POOR VISION

It is suggested that poor vision resulting from low dietary intakes of B12 might be reversed by taking supplements of the vitamin.

WHY TAKE THIS SUPPLEMENT?

With the exception of fermented soy, called tempeh, vitamin B12 is not found in plants, but is added to foods as a fortified ingredient. Strict vegetarians must take vitamin B12 to avoid deficiency, either as supplements or in fortified food. Pregnant and breastfeeding women may also benefit from supplements, along with people over 55 (the ability to absorb B12 declines with age). The following symptoms may also indicate a need for extra vitamin B12:

○ FATIGUE
○ POOR HAIR CONDITION
○ ECZEMA
○ DERMATITIS
○ SORE TONGUE
○ MEMORY LOSS
○ LACK OF CONCENTRATION
○ ANEMIA
○ IRRITABILITY
○ ANXIETY OR TENSION
○ TENDER OR SORE MUSCLES

EGGS
2.5mcg/4oz.

COD
2.0mcg/4oz.

BEEF
2.0mcg/4oz.

FORTIFIED BREAKFAST CEREALS
1.7mcg/4oz.

YEAST EXTRACT
0.5mcg/4oz.

FOLATE/FOLIC ACID

Prevents some birth defects ◆ May reduce the risk of heart disease ◆ Useful in treating megaloblastic anaemia

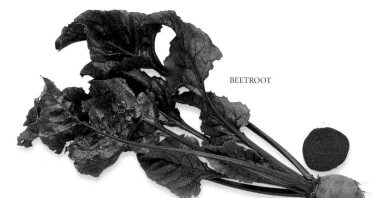

BEETROOT

CHEMICAL NAMES

- FOLIC ACID
- FOLACIN

PREPARATIONS

- TABLETS
- LIQUID
- CAPSULES

RDA FOR ADULTS

- 180/200MCG

HOW IT WORKS

Folate is found in foods such as black-eyed peas, beets, and wholegrain rice, bread, and pasta. Its synthetic form is folic acid, used in supplements and fortified foods such as cereal and yeast extract. It is better absorbed by the body than folate.

Folate is crucial for the correct development of a baby's spinal cord within the first three months of conception, so helping to prevent spina bifida. Folate is also vital for the proper formation of red blood cells, and appears to lower homocysteine levels which, when raised, seem to increase the risk of heart disease. Folate is also needed to break down protein for use by the body.

ABSORPTION HELPERS

Folate is best taken with food; B-complex vitamins, especially B12, help the body to absorb folate.

ABSORPTION INHIBITORS

Regular and large intakes of alcohol reduce folate

TOP SOURCES OF FOLATE mcg/4oz. of food

OX LIVER	FORTIFIED CEREAL	BLACK-EYED PEAS	BRUSSELS SPROUTS	PEANUTS
290mcg/4oz.	250mcg/4oz.	210mcg/4oz.	110mcg/4oz.	110mcg/4oz.

levels in the body, as can the painkiller aspirin, the contraceptive pill, and the drugs biguanides and metformin (used for the treatment of non-insulin dependent diabetes).

TAKING FOLIC ACID SUPPLEMENTS

The RDA for folate (180/200mg) is equivalent to three servings of fortified breakfast cereal. Women who wish to conceive, however, are encouraged to supplement their diet with 400mcg of folic acid daily. Upper safe levels of folate intake are 400mcg for prolonged use and 700mcg for short-term use. Optimum nutritionists recommend 400-1000mcg of folic acid daily.

PRECAUTIONS

High intakes of folic acid for a prolonged time may interfere with the body's absorption of the mineral zinc and can mask the deficiency of vitamin B12 in any blood samples taken from older people. People with epilepsy should seek advice from their doctor before supplementing because folic acid can affect and alter the action of epileptic drugs.

THERAPEUTIC USES

● HEART DISEASE

It may be possible to prevent seven percent of fatal male heart disease and five percent of female coronary-related deaths by taking folic acid.

● ANEMIA

The tiredness and fatigue caused by anemia (due to low intakes of folic acid) can be treated by taking folic acid supplements. Anemia during pregnancy can be treated with a combination of vitamin B12, folic acid, and iron.

● CERVICAL CANCER

Women taking the contraceptive pill who have reduced levels of folate in their blood may risk changes in cervical cells, which can lead to cancer. 10mg of folate daily can lead to significant improvements in cervical biopsies within three months.

● OSTEOPOROSIS

Homocysteine increases after menopause and interferes with bone formation, leading to osteoporosis. 5mg of folic acid a day may maintain bone strength and reduce the risk of osteoporosis by lowering levels of homocysteine.

● DEPRESSION

Raised homocysteine may increase the risk of low moods or depression. Lowering homocysteine with folic acid supplements may help to improve the symptoms.

WHY TAKE THIS SUPPLEMENT?

Women planning to conceive should take 400mcg of folic acid daily to reduce the risk of spina bifida. Men may also benefit from the same dosage to reduce the risk of atherosclerosis, caused by raised levels of homocysteine. People diagnosed with celiac disease, or on a poor diet, over 55, or consuming alcohol regularly may also benefit. Supplements could also be considered if the following symptoms occur:

○ TIREDNESS
○ FATIGUE
○ ECZEMA
○ CRACKED LIPS
○ ANXIETY AND TENSION
○ POOR MEMORY
○ POOR APPETITE
○ LOW MOODS
○ PALE SKIN

SPINACH
90mcg/4oz.

BROCCOLI
64mcg/4oz.

LETTUCE
55mcg/4oz.

GARBANZA BEANS
54mcg/4oz.

AVOCADO
11mcg/4oz.

VITAMIN C

Aids wound healing • Helps iron absorption • Anti-aging

May help to prevent cataracts

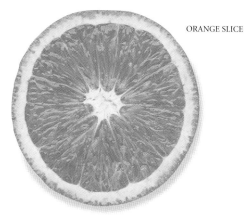

ORANGE SLICE

CHEMICAL NAMES

- ASCORBIC ACID

PREPARATIONS

- SOLID TABLETS
- TIMED-RELEASE TABLETS
- CHEWABLE TABLETS
- EFFERVESCENT TABLETS
- SYRUPS
- POWDERS

RDA FOR ADULTS

- 60MG

HOW IT WORKS

Vitamin C is essential for the body's production and maintenance of healthy collagen, which holds together cells in the skin, gums, and tendons. It also helps the white blood cells fight infection and is vital for the efficient healing of wounds. An antioxidant, vitamin C can help neutralize potential damaging free radicals that trigger aging and cancerous changes. It circulates in the blood, with any excess lost in the urine.

ABSORPTION HELPERS

Bioflavanoids *(see also p.89)*, which are found in fruits and vegetables enhance the absorption of vitamin C, which works best in conjunction with the minerals calcium and magnesium.

ABSORPTION INHIBITORS

Smoking, the contraceptive pill, the drug tetracyclin (for infections and acne), aspirin, and corticosteroid drugs (for treating rheumatoid arthritis) all reduce vitamin C levels.

TOP SOURCES OF VITAMIN C mg/4oz. of food

PAPAYA	GUAVA	BLACK-CURRANTS	GREEN PEPPER	BROCCOLI
60mg/4oz.	230mg/4oz.	200mg/4oz.	120mg/4oz.	87mg/4oz.

TAKING SUPPLEMENTS

The adult RDA for vitamin C (60mg) is equivalent to one glass of orange juice. The upper safe limit is considered to be 3000mg (3g) for short-term use and 2000mg (2g) for long-term use. Optimum nutritionists recommend daily intakes from 400-1000mg and therapeutic intakes of 1000mg-10,000mg (10g).

COMBINING SUPPLEMENTS

Have any ginseng supplements you might also be taking at least three hours before or after taking vitamin C or foods rich in vitamin C.

PRECAUTIONS

Megadoses of a gram a day or more may cause loose bowel movements, while those prone to kidney stones are advised against large intakes. Megadosing with vitamin C can also alter the results of blood and urine tests, and may mask blood in stools that can indicate bowel cancer, so first inform your doctor. People with diabetes must be aware that vitamin C in the urine can lead to inaccurate sugar results.

THERAPEUTIC USES

● CATARACTS

Taking vitamin C supplements has been found to reduce the risk of cataract development. People with cataracts have shown a marked improvement in vision within two weeks of taking a 350mg daily supplement in some cases.

● CANKER SORES

People with recurrent canker sores have remained free of outbreaks for over four years when taking 1,000-2,000mg (1-2g) vitamin C daily. Taking similar quantities at the first sign of symptoms may prevent full-blown outbreaks of canker sores.

● WOUND HEALING

People who take 200-250mg of vitamin C daily have an improved recovery rate after surgery, while the healing of bedsores and bleeding gums has been evident in people taking 250-500mg daily.

● INFECTIONS

Supplements of vitamin C may increase the immune system's ability to fight viral and bacterial infections, helping, for example, to reduce the duration of a cold.

WHY TAKE THIS SUPPLEMENT?

Smokers, who tend to have poor vitamin C intakes, have increased needs – estimated to be between 40mg a day to an extra 25mg with each cigarette. Infections, exposure to pollution (especially carbon monoxide), stress, people over 55, convalescents, athletes, and routine aspirin users may also benefit from vitamin C supplements. Optimum nutritionists believe that regular vitamin C supplements can not only treat specific problems, but can also help to prevent diseases such as cancer, heart disease, and infections. Signs that you may need a supplement include:

○ FREQUENT COLDS AND INFECTIONS
○ LACK OF ENERGY
○ BLEEDING, TENDER GUMS
○ EASY BRUISING
○ NOSE BLEEDS
○ SLOW WOUND HEALING
○ RED PIMPLES ON THE SKIN

STRAWBERRIES
77mg/4oz.

KIWI FRUIT
59mg/4oz.

ORANGES
54mg/4oz.

CABBAGE
49mg/4oz.

CAULIFLOWER
49mg/4oz.

VITAMIN D

Prevents rickets in infants ❖ Treats psoriasis ❖ May treat senile osteoporosis ❖ Prevents bone loss in periodontal disease

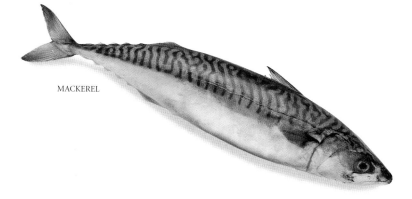

MACKEREL

CHEMICAL NAMES

- CHOLECALCIFEROL
- CALCIFEROL
- ERGOSTEROL

PREPARATIONS

- COD LIVER OIL
- CAPSULES
- TABLETS
- LIQUID

RDA FOR ADULTS

- 5MCG

HOW IT WORKS

Vitamin D acts like a hormone, meaning that it is formed in one place but carries out its function in another part of the body. Most of the vitamin D used in the body is formed under the skin through exposure to the sun; ultra-violet rays change it from an inactive form into an active form. Vitamin D is also crucial for encouraging the absorption of calcium from food. It directly increases the rate of mineral deposits on bones. Without enough of it, the body cannot build or maintain strong bones.

ABSORPTION HELPERS

The known dietary sources of vitamin D (see below) tend to contain fats or oils, which enhance its absorption.

ABSORPTION INHIBITORS

Cholestyramine, which is used in the treatment of high cholesterol, and mineral oil, which is used as a laxative, both reduce levels of absorption.

TOP SOURCES OF VITAMIN D mcg/4oz. of food

COD LIVER OIL	HERRING	MACKEREL	SARDINES	RAINBOW TROUT
210mcg/4oz.	19mcg/4oz.	18mcg/4oz.	11mcg/4oz.	10.6mcg/4oz.

TAKING SUPPLEMENTS

The adult RDA for vitamin D (5mcg) can be obtained by eating just two canned sardines in tomato sauce. It is recommended that those people who are over the age of 65 should consume 10mcg supplements of vitamin D per day if their diet is poor in vitamin D sources. The upper safe intake for the long term is 10mcg per day, and 50mcg per day in the short term. Optimum nutritionists recommend that adults should all consume between 10–20mcg per day, and take 10–25 mcg per day for therapeutic reasons.

PRECAUTIONS

Infants are most at risk of overdosing on vitamin D, so supplementation must be undertaken only on medical advice. Taking vitamin D-rich cod liver oil plus vitamin D supplements could result in excessive intakes.

THERAPEUTIC USES

● **BREASTFEEDING**
Young babies could be at risk of developing soft, rickety bones, which bend and bow if there are low levels of vitamin D in their mother's breast milk. This is usually due to the mother eating a poor diet and having little exposure to sunlight. Breastfeeding mothers who take 10mcg per day of vitamin D supplements can avoid this problem.

● **OSTEOPOROSIS**
By taking vitamin D supplements daily, elderly people and those at risk of developing osteoporosis may help to increase the beneficial effects of calcium absorption by the body to help strengthen bones and prevent any brittleness from developing.

● **PERIODONTAL DISEASE**
People with weak gum tissue may benefit from taking vitamin D supplements daily in order to help reduce any further loss of their jawbone from periodontal disease.

● **PSORIASIS**
Those people who suffer from psoriasis may find that they also have low levels of vitamin D. The symptoms of this skin condition may improve if psoriasis sufferers increase their daily dietary intakes of vitamin D.

WHY TAKE THIS SUPPLEMENT?

Anyone who has limited exposure to sunshine during the summer months, some vegetarians and vegans, older people over 55, pregnant and breastfeeding women, young children, and those concerned about developing osteoporosis may all benefit from taking vitamin D supplements daily. Asian women and children are also advised to take supplements if they are vegetarian, have low intakes of calcium, and their skin has limited exposure to sunlight. Signs of a lack of vitamin D – either through a poor diet and/or from poor exposure to sunlight – include:

❍ POOR GROWTH
❍ BONE DEFORMITIES
❍ RICKETS
❍ OSTEOMALACIA
❍ BONE PAIN
❍ MUSCLE WEAKNESS
❍ CONSTIPATION

SALMON
8.0mcg/4oz.

MARGARINE
7.9mcg/4oz.

FRESH TUNA
7.2mcg/4oz.

EGGS
1.75mcg/4oz.

CHEDDAR CHEESE
0.26mcg/4oz.

VITAMIN E

May reduce the risk of heart disease • May help lower the risk of cancer

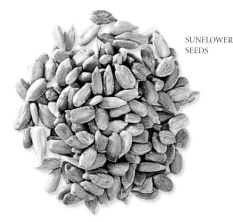

SUNFLOWER SEEDS

CHEMICAL NAMES

- TOCOPHEROL; ALPHA, BETA, GAMMA, AND DELTA

PREPARATIONS

- CAPSULES
- TABLETS
- LIQUID
- OIL
- SOFTGEL CAPSULES

RDA FOR ADULTS

- 8/10MG

HOW IT WORKS

Vitamin E is an anti-oxidant vitamin, helping to neutralize potentially damaging free radicals in the body. It is particularly important for helping to keep cell walls in good condition and for the healthy maintenance of the skin, nerves, muscles, red blood cells, body circulation, and heart. Vitamin E improves the activity of vitamin A in the body, and, unlike other fat-soluble vitamins, seems to be stored for only a short time in the body – indicating the need for very regular intakes.

ABSORPTION HELPERS

Vitamin C and selenium help the action of vitamin E in the body.

ABSORPTION INHIBITORS

The drug cholestyramine, taken to reduce raised cholesterol levels, inhibits absorption of vitamin E. Excess intakes of iron, copper, and manganese can all reduce vitamin E in the body, as can

TOP SOURCES OF VITAMIN E mg/100g of food

WHEATGERM OIL	SUNFLOWER SEED OIL	SUNFLOWER SEEDS	FILBERTS	ALMONDS
137mg/100g	49mg/100g	37mg/100g	25mg/100g	24mg/100g

trans-fats in some margarine and processed food, air pollution, and the contraceptive pill.

TAKING VITAMIN E SUPPLEMENTS

The RDA for vitamin E (8/10mg) is equivalent to 1oz. of sunflower seeds. The most effective supplement form of vitamin E is d-alpha tocopherol; avoid dl-alpha tocopherol, which is not as effective. The safe upper limit, showing no short or long term adverse effects, is 800mg a day. Optimum nutritionists recommend 100–1000mg a day for adults as a preventive and therapeutic dose.

COMBINING SUPPLEMENTS

Products with 25mcg of selenium for each 200mg of vitamin E will increase its potency. Take any supplements containing iron at least eight hours before or after vitamin E supplements to avoid vitamin E destruction.

PRECAUTIONS

When taken by people with vitamin K deficiency, high intakes of vitamin E can adversely affect blood-clotting mechanisms. People with high blood pressure, rheumatic heart disease, or ischemic heart disease should take high intakes only under close medical supervision.

THERAPEUTIC USES

● **HEART DISEASE**
Vitamin E supplements of 80–100g may lower the risk of heart disease, stroke, and angina by reducing the formation of atherosclerosis plaques on artery walls.

● **CANCER**
Good intakes of vitamin E may help protect against some forms of cancer, especially of the lung and the cervix.

● **CATARACTS**
People who take vitamin E supplements may have a lower incidence of developing cataracts.

● **INFECTIONS**
Vitamin E supplements may enhance the action of the immune system to fight infection.

● **OSTEOARTHRITIS**
Vitamin E may help to relieve the pain associated with osteoarthritis, possibly through its action as an anti-inflammatory agent.

● **MALE FERTILITY**
Intakes of 600mg of vitamin E daily have been shown to significantly benefit sperm numbers and also help to improve male fertility.

WHY TAKE THIS SUPPLEMENT?

People with a diet high in polyun-saturated fats that includes a high proportion of margarine, vegetable oils, nuts, and seeds, may need vitamin E supplements as much as people who cannot absorb fat. Vitamin E may also be appropriate for people with a family history of heart disease, those exposed to pollution, and anyone interested in slowing down the aging process. The following signs may also indicate a need for this supplement:

○ EXHAUSTION AFTER LIGHT EXERCISE
○ EASY BRUISING
○ SLOW WOUND HEALING
○ VARICOSE VEINS
○ LOSS OF MUSCLE TONE
○ LACK OF SEX DRIVE
○ INFERTILITY

PINOLA
14mg/100g

SWEET POTATO
4mg/100g

AVOCADO
3mg/100g

GRANOLA
3mg/100g

SPINACH
2mg/100g

VITAMIN H/BIOTIN

Can help with diabetes ⬦ Improves eczema and dermatitis ⬦ May help weight loss

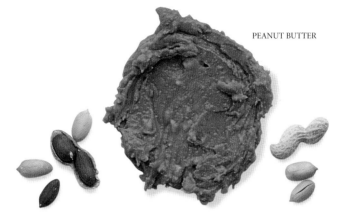

PEANUT BUTTER

CHEMICAL NAMES

- BIOTIN
- D-BIOTIN

PREPARATIONS

- CAPSULES
- TABLETS

RDA FOR ADULTS

- 150MCG

HOW IT WORKS

Biotin works alongside other B vitamins, helping the body burn proteins, carbohydrates, and fats in the diet and turn them into energy for the body's cells to utilize. Biotin also has a particularly important role to play in the production of fatty acids, which ensure the health of the skin, nerves, and hair, as well as many other functions throughout the body. It is also said to help prevent hair from turning gray.

ABSORPTION HELPERS

Other B vitamins and the minerals magnesium and manganese aid biotin's absorption. Supplements containing biotin are best taken with meals.

ABSORPTION INHIBITORS

A substance called avidin, which is found in raw egg white, binds itself to biotin and prevents its absorption, although this blockage is cancelled out during the cooking process. Absorption is also reduced by regular

TOP SOURCES OF VITAMIN H mcg/4oz. of food

DRY ROASTED PEANUTS
130mcg/4oz.

CRUNCHY PEANUT BUTTER
102mcg/4oz.

FILBERTS
76mcg/4oz.

ALMONDS
64mcg/4oz.

PORK KIDNEY
53mcg/4oz.

intakes of alcohol, which lowers the levels of biotin in the bloodstream.

TAKING BIOTIN SUPPLEMENTS

The RDA for biotin (150mcg) is easily met through a mixed diet; the body's need for biotin is very small, and supplements are only needed in certain cases. Intakes of 2500mcg (2.5g) are considered to be the safe upper limit for long- and short-term use. Optimum nutritionists recommend 50–200mcg a day of biotin for both general and therapeutic uses.

PRECAUTIONS

No adverse effects have been found from high intakes of biotin.

THERAPEUTIC USES

● DIABETES

There is a small amount of evidence to suggest that biotin may work with insulin to reduce blood sugar levels, and biotin supplements may be beneficial in diabetic peripheral neuropathy – where damage to the nerves in the hands and feet leads to numbness and loss of sensation.

● WEIGHT LOSS

It has been claimed that as biotin has a role in fat metabolism, so perhaps it may aid weight loss.

● ECZEMA AND DERMATITIS

It has been suggested that eczema and dermatitis are alleviated by taking biotin supplements and that biotin may improve dermatitis in infants.

● GRAYING

While there is no scientific evidence to support the claim, it has been noted that people say that regular supplementation with biotin helps to stop hair from turning gray.

● INTESTINAL PROBLEMS

Biotin supplements may be useful for anyone who has difficulty with intestinal absorption, and also for those with kidney problems, which can result in losses of biotin through the urine.

● TUBE FEEDING

Patients fed long-term on parenteral nutrition (when nutrients are delivered via a line into the veins) can be at risk of biotin deficiency and may need extra biotin in their formulation.

WHY TAKE THIS SUPPLEMENT?

Those people taking antibiotics and sulfonamide anti-bacterial drugs may benefit from biotin supplements. People with diabetes may find that daily biotin supplements can help support the breakdown of fat and carbohydrate; it could also prove useful to people over 55. However, biotin is widely found in foods and is manufactured by the body in the gut. The following symptoms are typical of a lack of biotin in the diet and may signal a need to improve intakes:

- SCALY, DRY SKIN AROUND NOSE AND MOUTH
- PATCHES OF HAIR LOSS AND REVERSIBLE BALDNESS
- BRITTLE HAIR
- LOSS OF APPETITE
- MUSCLE PAINS AND WASTING
- NAUSEA
- HALLUCINATIONS
- TIREDNESS
- DEPRESSION

EGG YOLK
50mcg/4oz.

OX LIVER
50mcg/4oz.

WALNUTS
19mcg/4oz.

SESAME SEEDS
11mcg/4oz.

COTTAGE CHEESE
3mcg/4oz.

VITAMIN K

May improve bone strength in osteoporosis ◆ May reduce symptoms of vomiting and nausea in pregnancy

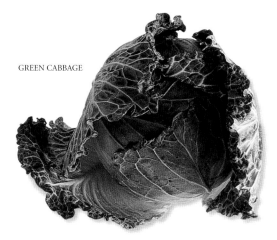

GREEN CABBAGE

CHEMICAL NAMES

- PHYTONADIONE
  MENADIOL

PREPARATIONS

- TABLETS
- LIQUIDS

RDA FOR ADULTS

- 65/80MCG

HOW IT WORKS

Bacteria make vitamin K in the colon, from where it is absorbed back across the colon wall into the bloodstream to become one of several of blood-clotting factors. It is also needed for the production of proteins that help to keep teeth and bones healthy and strong.

ABSORPTION HELPERS

Probiotic foods, such as yogurt containing "live" bacteria, can help promote the growth of good bacteria in the colon and enhance vitamin K production in the body.

ABSORPTION INHIBITORS

Cholestyramine, a drug taken for the treatment of raised cholesterol levels, and aspirin, taken for pain relief, can both reduce the absorption of vitamin K in the body. Antibiotics, taken to kill disease-causing bacteria, actually kill all bacteria, whether good or bad. They also kill vitamin K bacteria by synthesizing them.

TOP SOURCES OF VITAMIN K (no figures available)

BROCCOLI

BRUSSELS
SPROUTS

GREEN
CABBAGE

YOGURT

ALFALFA

TAKING VITAMIN K SUPPLEMENTS

The RDA (65/80mcg) was only set in 1989. Humans make a substantial part of their vitamin K requirement in the colon, and vitamin K is present in the diet, supplied by the equivalent of a serving of Brussels sprouts.

PRECAUTIONS

Megadoses of vitamin K should be avoided as they can build up, causing the breakdown of red blood cells. While some blood-thinning drugs can inhibit the absorption of natural vitamin K, synthetic K in supplement form can counteract its effectiveness and is therefore best avoided. Large doses of vitamin K may lead to liver damage and problems such as jaundice in infants and children.

THERAPEUTIC USES

● OSTEOPOROSIS

Vitamin K levels have been found to be low in some women with osteoporosis, which increases the risk of bone fractures in later life. Vitamin K is needed for the bone-strengthening mineral calcium to be deposited on the bone structure. It is possible that where vitamin K levels are low, supplements may help to improve bone strength and reduce the risk of fractures.

● HEAVY BLOOD LOSS

Women who experience a heavy loss of blood during menstruation could benefit from a supplement of vitamin K, which may help to reduce the flow of blood.

● MENOPAUSAL WOMEN

Vitamin K given to healthy postmenopausal women has been shown to reduce losses of calcium in the urine and improve the calcium-binding properties of the hormone, which lays calcium onto bones.

● PREGNANCY

Low vitamin K levels have been recorded in pregnant women suffering from nausea and vomiting. Supplements of 5mg a day plus 25mg vitamin C daily has been shown to give relief within 72 hours.

● BABIES

Giving supplements to babies with low levels of vitamin K can help establish good blood-clotting mechanisms and reduce the risk of bleeding.

WHY TAKE THIS SUPPLEMENT?

The drug warfarin, prescribed to regulate blood clotting, stops bacterial production of vitamin K in the colon and could increase dietary requirements if it is taken in the long term. All newborn babies are given vitamin K either as supplements or in form of an injection in order to improve their blood clotting abilities. People who suffer from malabsorption problems, such as celiac disease, colitis, and Crohn's disease, may also benefit from vitamin K supplements, as could women who experience excessive menstrual bleeding and people who have undergone surgery. Signs that you may need a vitamin K supplement include:

- ○ EXCESSIVE DIARRHEA
- ○ EASY BLEEDING
- ○ BLEEDING THAT IS SLOW TO STOP

EGG YOLK

SAFFLOWER OIL

SOYBEAN OIL

FISH LIVER OIL

KELP

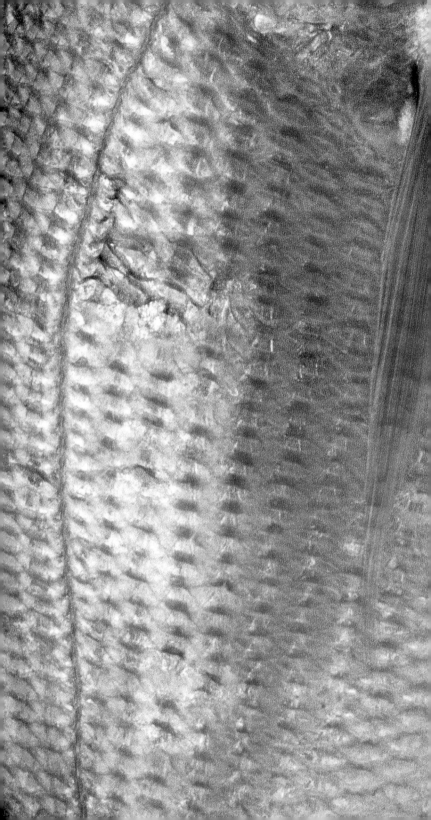

Guide to Minerals

Minerals are inorganic substances found in rocks and ore, some of which are essential to human life, that enter our diets via plants and animals that have fed on these plants. This guide charts the vital functions that minerals play in the body.

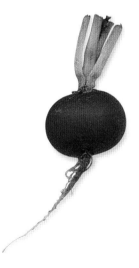

CALCIUM

Helps maximize bone density in teenagers ✦ Reduces risk of osteoporosis ✦ Relieves leg cramps ✦ May improve PMS

LOW-FAT
COW'S MILK

CHEMICAL NAMES

- CALCIUM CARBONATE
- CALCIUM MALATE
- CALCIUM GLUCONATE
- CALCIUM PHOSPHATE
- CALCIUM CITRATE
- CALCIUM CITRATE
  MALATE

PREPARATIONS

- TABLETS
- CAPSULES
- SOFTGEL CAPSULES
- POWDER

RDA/DRI

- 1000MG

HOW IT WORKS

About 99 percent of the body's calcium is found in the bones and teeth, where it is crucial for building and maintaining strength. The other one percent is present in body tissues and fluids, where it is involved in muscle contraction and blood clotting.

ABSORPTION HELPERS

Vitamin D is vital for the effective absorption of calcium. There is evidence that the essential fatty acids found in evening primrose oil and fish oil also improve the body's uptake of calcium from food and drink.

ABSORPTION INHIBITORS

Phytate, a type of fiber found in spinach, dried legumes, some nuts, and wholegrain cereals, may bind with calcium in the digestive system to create unabsorbable substances. Oxalates, which are present in rhubarb, have a similar effect. Large intakes of the mineral magnesium and too

TOP SOURCES OF CALCIUM mg/4oz. of food

EDAM
770mg/4oz.

CHEDDAR
CHEESE
720mg/4oz.

SESAME SEEDS
670mg/4oz.

SARDINES IN
OIL
550mg/4oz.

STEAMED TOFU
510mg/4oz.

much phosphorus from cola drinks can also upset the balance of calcium in the body.

TAKING CALCIUM SUPPLEMENTS

The adult RDA/DRI for calcium (1000mg) is equivalent to a small can of sardines with bones, plus half a pint of low-fat milk. The best-absorbed forms are thought to be calcium amino acid chelate or calcium citrate, which has twice the absorption rate of calcium carbonate. Supplements taken at night or combined with fish oil and evening primrose oil may increase the chances of calcium being laid onto bone, with the oils also helping to reduce calcium losses in the urine. The National Osteoporosis Society and optimum nutritionists suggest intakes should be higher than the RDA, with levels of 1,500mg advised. The safe upper level for long-term usage is 1,500mg, 1,900mg for short-term usage.

COMBINING SUPPLEMENTS

Calcium supplements are available with added vitamin D to help provide optimum absorption.

PRECAUTIONS

The body regulates the level of calcium closely, so if long-term usage remains at 1,500mg a day excessive accumulation in blood or tissues is unlikely. Large intakes over a prolonged time, however, may lead to calcium being deposited in the kidneys and on artery walls, resulting in blocked arteries and kidney stones.

THERAPEUTIC USES

● OSTEOPOROSIS

Increasing calcium intakes by 800mg a day has been shown to improve the bone density of teenage girls. It is possible that these dosages could help to strengthen bones during this critical growth period, making bones stronger for life and reducing the risk of osteoporosis, which increases the incidence of bone fracture in later life.

● REDUCTION OF BONE LOSS IN OLDER WOMEN

It has been proven that 400mg supplements daily help reduce bone loss in postmenopausal women.

● PREMENSTRUAL SYNDROME

There is evidence that calcium supplements,

taken with magnesium, help relieve premenstrual pains. Water retention may also improve with 1,000mg of calcium daily.

● LEG CRAMPS

A 600mg supplement taken at night may help to improve leg cramps. Up to 1,000mg daily can also benefit leg cramps associated with pregnancy.

WHY TAKE THIS SUPPLEMENT?

Children and teen-agers who eat few dairy-based foods may have lower than recommended intakes of calcium and could benefit from taking supplements. People on restricted diets that avoid dairy foods or weight-reducing diets, vegans, and women concerned about reducing the risk of osteoporosis in later life, may also need supplements. Signs also include:

○ MUSCLE ACHES AND PAINS
○ MUSCLE TWITCHING
○ MUSCLE SPASMS
○ MUSCLE CRAMPS
○ POOR BONE DENSITY FOR AGE

DRIED FIGS
250mg/4oz.

FRUIT YOGURT
150mg/4oz.

WHOLE MILK
115mg/4oz.

GRANOLA
110mg/4oz.

GREEN BEANS
33mg/4oz.

CHROMIUM

Improves blood sugar control ✦ May influence
cholesterol levels ✦ Popular in weight-control supplements

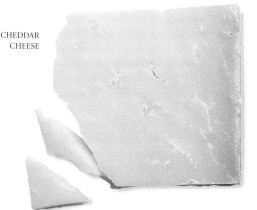

CHEDDAR
CHEESE

CHEMICAL NAMES

- CHROMIUM PICOLINATE
- CHROMIUM
  POLYNICOTINATE

PREPARATIONS

- CAPSULES
- TABLETS
- VEGETARIAN CAPSULES
- BREWER'S YEAST
- LIQUID

RDA FOR ADULTS

- 50–200MG

HOW IT WORKS

Chromium appears to
increase the action of the
hormone insulin in the
body. Insulin controls levels
of sugar in the blood and
plays a role in fat storage.
Chromium may help
people with diabetes
control their blood sugar
and help generally with
weight loss.

ABSORPTION HELPERS

The three amino acids
(glycine, glutamic acid, and
cystine) and niacin (vitamin B) help absorption.

ABSORPTION
INHIBITORS

Additives and pesticides
are thought to lower
chromium levels in the
body, while diets high in
sugar may increase losses
of chromium in the urine.

TAKING
CHROMIUM
SUPPLEMENTS

A trace mineral, chromium
should be administered
with great care. A safe
level of intake is believed
to be 50mcg per day for
adults, and 0.1–1.0mcg

TOP SOURCES OF CHROMIUM (figures not available)

BREWER'S
YEAST

MEAT

WHOLEGRAINS

BLACK-EYED
PEAS

NUTS

per kilogram (2.2lb) per day for adolescents and children. Safe upper limits of 200mcg daily for long-term usage and 300mcg for short-term use are advised. Optimum nutritionists recommend intakes of 100mcg a day for adults, rising up to levels of 200mcg a day for therapeutic uses. Chromium picolinate, chromium polynicotinate, trivalent chromium, and brewer's yeast are thought to be the best supplements.

PRECAUTIONS

Chromium is toxic only if intakes of several grams a day are consumed.

THERAPEUTIC USES

● CHOLESTEROL LOWERING

Chromium levels may be low in people with blocked arteries, which can lead to heart disease. Research on people with raised blood cholesterol taking 200mcg of chromium tripicolinate daily showed evidence of reduced levels of LDL or "bad" cholesterol.

● DIABETES

People with diabetes frequently have blood sugar levels higher than normal, which can lead to complications in later life such as damage to nerves in the hands and feet, atherosclerosis and heart disease, and poor vision. Limited research indicates that blood sugar levels can be reduced by an average of 18 percent if 200mcg of chromium tripicolinate is taken daily.

● HYPOGLYCEMIA

Hypoglycemia (low blood sugar levels), which can cause symptoms such as anxiety, over-excitement, and sweats, has been successfully treated in a group of women who took 200mcg chromium daily. The extra chromium may help correct either a shortage of chromium in the diet, or an inability to metabolize this mineral.

● GLAUCOMA

Glaucoma – in which raised pressure in the eye causes blind spots and eventual blindness – has revealed a tendency for low blood levels of chromium. Supplements may be helpful.

● FOOD CRAVINGS

Anecdotal evidence suggests that raising chromium intakes can help reduce sweet cravings and hunger, and so help weight reduction.

WHY TAKE THIS SUPPLEMENT?

Older people over 55 years of age and people who exercise regularly may have increased losses of chromium, while those suffering stress and trauma appear to have decreased levels. People who eat diets rich in processed foods containing few good chromium sources, or with a poor ability to balance blood sugar levels in their body and who have a tendency to gain weight, may also benefit from supplements. Other symptoms of a lack of chromium in the body can include:

○ POOR BLOOD SUGAR CONTROL
○ DIZZINESS AND IRRITABILITY AFTER SIX HOURS WITHOUT FOOD
○ NEED FOR FREQUENT MEALS
○ FEELING SLEEPY
○ EXCESSIVE THIRST
○ STRONG DESIRE FOR SWEET FOODS
○ RAISED BLOOD FATS

RED KIDNEY BEANS

MUNG BEANS

ADUKI BEANS

PEAS

PEANUTS

COPPER

Can help to lower cholesterol ● Lowers risk of osteoporosis

Reduces pain of arthritis

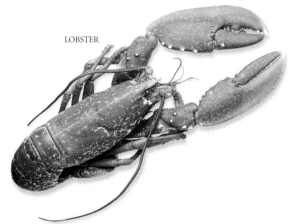

LOBSTER

CHEMICAL NAMES

- COPPER PICOLINATE
- COPPER ASPARTATE
- COPPER CITRATE

PREPARATIONS

- TABLETS
- CAPSULES

RDA FOR ADULTS

- 1.5–3MG

HOW IT WORKS

While copper has no one specific role in the body, it is needed to facilitate a wide variety of actions. It is needed, for example, for the body's conversion of the mineral iron into the oxygen-carrying pigment called hemoglobin, and for making the amino acid tyrosine, which is involved in forming the color of hair and skin. It plays a role in the action of various proteins needed for growth, to aid the proper workings of the nerves, and in the release of energy. Copper also has an important role in the control of inflammation.

ABSORPTION HELPERS

Copper is generally well-absorbed by the body (although less so with increasing age). Vegetarian diets provide lower levels of copper.

ABSORPTION INHIBITORS

Too much zinc can upset the balance of copper, as can long-term use of antacid indigestion remedies.

TOP SOURCES OF COPPER mg/4oz. of food

CALVES' LIVER	OYSTERS	SARDINES IN TOMATO SAUCE	SUNFLOWER SEEDS	CRAB
11mg/4oz.	7.5mg/4oz.	2.4mg/4oz.	2.27mg/4oz.	1.77mg/4oz.

TAKING COPPER SUPPLEMENTS

Copper is another trace mineral, and we should aim to consume 1.5mg of copper daily, equivalent to eating 3oz. of sardines. Optimum nutritionists suggest 2mg a day is required and 5mg daily can be taken to correct a deficiency, although in practice deficiency is quite rare. Copper is often found in multimineral supplements at levels of 1–2mg. The most easily absorbed forms of copper are copper amino acid chelate and gluconate, while copper sulfate and copper nitrate are also readily absorbed into the body's bloodstream.

PRECAUTIONS

Copper may trigger migraines in susceptible people. Excessive intakes of copper are rare, although they are possible if water is drunk from contaminated copper pipes. Copper toxicity can lead to vomiting and diarrhea, the accumulation of copper in the liver, schizophrenia, osteoporosis, and bone fractures. Large intakes of copper can also reduce the body's stores of the mineral manganese.

THERAPEUTIC USES

● HEART PROBLEMS
Low intakes of copper may be associated with increased LDL "bad" cholesterol and decreased HDL "good" cholesterol. This may account for low copper levels being a potential contributing factor in heart and circulatory problems, which may lead to full-blown heart disease.

● INFECTIONS
A lack of copper in the diet may lower the body's immune system. Normal intakes may help to reduce the risk of infection.

● OSTEOPOROSIS
Blood levels of copper are thought to be directly associated with bone mass density; even a mild deficiency of copper may trigger, then worsen, osteo-porotic lesions in bones. Boosting poor dietary intakes may help reduce the risk of osteoporosis.

● ARTHRITIS
Short-term treatment with copper salicylates has been shown to reduce fever and swelling, and to increase joint mobility in those who suffer from rheumatoid arthritis.

WHY TAKE THIS SUPPLEMENT?

While copper is found to be rarely deficient in the diet (with some being provided through the copper which dissolves from copper water pipes and cooking pans), people over 55 and those taking high dosage zinc supplements may require a modest supplement of copper. Premature babies and those babies who might be wrongly fed with unmodified cow's milk may also need additional copper supplements, but such action should only be taken on the advice of a doctor. Poor intakes of copper can lead to the following range of symptoms:
- ○ FAILURE OF BABIES TO FEED AND GROW
- ○ IRON-DEFICIENCY ANEMIA
- ○ TIREDNESS
- ○ CHANGES TO HAIR COLOR
- ○ CHANGES TO SKIN PIGMENTATION

LOBSTER
1.35mg/4oz.

PEANUTS
1.2mg/4oz.

MUSHROOMS
0.4mg/4oz.

WHOLEWHEAT BREAD
0.26mg/4oz.

PRUNES
0.14mg/4oz.

FLUORIDE

May help reduce the risk of tooth decay

May help to strengthen bones

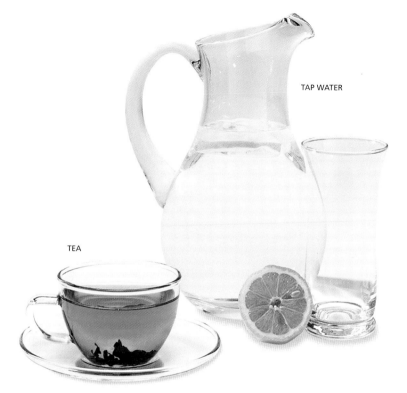

TAP WATER

TEA

CHEMICAL NAMES

- SODIUM FLUORIDE
- CALCIUM FLUORIDE

PREPARATIONS

- NOT USUALLY FOUND IN MULTIMINERAL SUPPLEMENTS

RDA FOR ADULTS

- 1.5–4MG

HOW IT WORKS

The main use of fluoride in the body is in the hardening of both bones and tooth enamel. When it is incorporated into the teeth as they are forming, fluoride helps prevent tooth decay and appears to reduce the risk of decay once the teeth have erupted from the gum. It is estimated that adults consume around 1.8mg fluoride per day, with 25 percent of this coming from food, and 70 percent of the remaining amount from drinking tea, coffee, and other drinks containing tap water. Fluoride intakes increase to approximately 2.9 mg a day in areas where the tap water is fluoridated, assuming a daily consumption of 2 pints of water. A safe upper limit for infants and children has been set at 0.025mg per pound per day.

Cooking in fluorinated water raises the levels of this mineral in many foods.

ABSORPTION HELPERS

The minerals phosphate and sulfate increase the uptake of fluoride and aid its absorption more effectively into the body.

ABSORPTION INHIBITORS

The minerals magnesium, calcium, and aluminum all seem to lower the body's ability to take up fluoride. Long-term use of antacid tablets containing aluminum, which are taken to reduce acid indigestion, may also lower fluoride levels.

TAKING FLUORIDE SUPPLEMENTS

Oral fluoride tablets have been claimed to help reduce dental decay in children, but should only be taken under super-vision and on the specific advice of either a dentist or doctor. Mouth rinses and toothpaste with added fluoride also contribute to daily intakes, especially when swallowed instead of – as is intended – being spat out. Most fluoride in the diet comes from drinking tea, coffee, and water, with foods such as fish eaten together with their bones supplying only a quarter of the daily fluoride intake.

PRECAUTIONS

Fluorosis is the name given to fluoride toxicity in the body. Chalky white patches on the surface of the teeth, known as mottling, are a clear sign of excess intakes of fluoride in the diet. This usually affects children in areas where the water supply is fluoridated and extra fluoride is also taken in via other sources such as swallowed fluoridated toothpastes and mouth rinses. Adults can also be badly affected by high intakes, with 0.5–2.6g a day over a short time leading to depression and potentially fatal fluorisis. Fluoride offers protection against decay by strengthening tooth enamel and reducing the risk of acid erosion.

THERAPEUTIC USES

● **DENTAL DECAY**

Drinking fluoridated water from birth is said to give maximum protection against tooth decay. There have been some reports that drinking tea also helps to lower the incidence of tooth decay, although adding sugar to tea could inhibit the beneficial effects of this drink.

● **OSTEOPOROSIS**

Osteoporosis has been reported to be less frequent in people who live in areas with high fluoride levels, suggesting that it may have a possible role to play in helping to control the development of this bone-thinning condition. Fluoride supplements are currently being investigated, with scientists suggesting that this nutrient may protect the bones from thinning and actually maintain their density.

● **INNER EAR**

The formation of new bone in the inner part of the ear is a common cause of worsening deafness as people age. It has been suggested that treating such conditions with six 16mg of sodium fluoride supplements under medical supervision may actually help stabilize the progression of bone growth in the ear and the associated deafness that results from it.

WHY TAKE THIS SUPPLEMENT?

Supplementation with fluoride tablets is only advisable after consultation with a doctor or dentist. If you have children and live in an area where the water is not fluoridated, however, you may want to consider asking your dentist about supplements. Signs of deficiency, although rare, include:

❍ BADLY FORMED TOOTH ENAMEL
❍ BRITTLE BONES

IRON

Reduces tiredness and fatigue ◆ Improves concentration

Provides relief from painful periods ◆ Restores skin tone

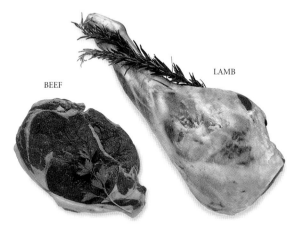

LAMB

BEEF

CHEMICAL NAMES

- FERROUS SULFATE
- FERROUS GLUCONATE
- FERROUS FUMARATE
- FERROUS PEPTONATE
- FERRIC CITRATE

PREPARATIONS

- TABLETS
- CAPSULES
- LIQUID
- SOFTGEL CAPSULES

RDA FOR ADULTS

- 10–15MG

HOW IT WORKS

Iron forms part of the red pigment, hemoglobin, in blood, which gives blood its color and helps to transport oxygen around the body to all cells. Two-thirds of the body's total store of iron is present in hemoglobin; the remainder can be found in the liver, spleen, bone marrow, and muscles.

ABSORPTION HELPERS

The fruit sugar fructose and also vitamin C help the iron found in plant sources, such as nuts and seeds, to be absorbed effectively into the body.

ABSORPTION INHIBITORS

Tannin in tea, which gives the drink its astringent taste, can bind with iron and reduce its absorption via the digestive system into the blood. The fibrous phytate substances in cereals, especially bran, and spinach have a similar effect, as can excess intakes of calcium. A particular type of protein found in eggs, and the tannic acid

TOP SOURCES OF IRON mg/4oz. of food

BRANFLAKES	ALL-BRAN	SESAME SEEDS	BAKED VENISON	SARDINES IN TOMATO SAUCE
20mg/4oz.	12mg/4oz.	10.4mg/4oz.	7.8mg/4oz.	4.6mg/4oz.

found in the supplement St. John's wort (taken to lift low moods; *see also p.111*), may also reduce the absorption of iron, as can the antacids found in indigestion remedies and the drug tetracycline, which is prescribed for infections and acne.

TAKING IRON SUPPLEMENTS

The adult RDA for iron (10–15mg) is equivalent to one bowl of iron-fortified breakfast cereal, a handful of dried apricots, and a steak. Optimum nutritionists recommend 15mg a day, rising to 25mg for treating symptoms of iron deficiency such as anemia. While short-term use of 80mg will not cause harm, the safe upper limit for continued use is set at 15mg. The ferrous sulfate form of iron is believed to increase the risk of constipation in people sensitive to this problem. Supplements containing organic iron, such as ferrous gluconate, ferrous fumerate, ferrous citrate, or ferrous peptonate, are absorbed best by the body.

PRECAUTIONS

Prolonged high intakes of iron can be harmful to young children especially.

High levels in adults seem to result in accelerated aging and the possibly increased risk of heart disease and infection. Intakes of 10,000mg (100g) are lethal.

THERAPEUTIC USES

● IRON DEFICIENCY ANEMIA

If iron-deficiency anemia is diagnosed, a medical practitioner usually prescribes treatment with iron supplements.

● IMPROVED CONCENTRATION

It has been suggested that supplementing with the RDA could improve academic performance, particularly in young teenage girls with poor dietary iron intakes.

● PAINFUL PERIODS

Early evidence suggests that taking daily supplements of iron may help to ease the pain often associated with monthly menstruation.

● FATIGUE

Tiredness and fatigue associated with poor intakes of iron in the diet can be improved by taking supplements of iron at RDA levels.

WHY TAKE THIS SUPPLEMENT?

Women who are trying to conceive may benefit from taking iron supplements, especially if their diet supplies little or no meat and their pregnancies are close together. Vegetarians, vegans, athletes, and those who have undergone surgery may also benefit from iron supplements, as could some elderly people who exist on a nutritionally restricted diet and drink large quantities of tea. Signs of needing extra iron include:

- ○ TIREDNESS
- ○ FATIGUE
- ○ POOR CONCENTRATION
- ○ HEADACHES
- ○ HAIR LOSS
- ○ SHORTAGE OF BREATH
- ○ BRITTLE, RIDGED, BREAKABLE NAILS
- ○ PALE COMPLEXION
- ○ LOSS OF APPETITE
- ○ REPEATED INFECTIONS

DRIED APRICOTS
3.4mg/4oz.

BROILED RUMP STEAK
3.4mg/4oz.

CANNED CRAB
2.8mg/4oz.

TUNA IN OIL
1.6mg/4oz.

BAKED LAMB
1.5mg/4oz.

IODINE

Reduces swollen thyroid gland ❖ May relieve painful breasts ❖ May reduce risk of breast cancer

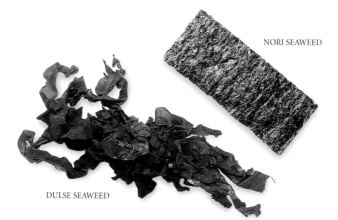

NORI SEAWEED

DULSE SEAWEED

CHEMICAL NAMES

- IODINE

PREPARATIONS

- CAPSULES
- TABLETS
- LIQUID
- KELP

RDA FOR ADULTS

- 150MCG

HOW IT WORKS

Approximately 64 percent of iodine – which amounts to about 8mg of iodine in total – is located in the thyroid gland in the neck, where it is used to make the two thyroid hormones tri-iodothyronine and thyroxine. These hormones regulate the speed of the body's metabolism, including the rate at which calories are burned. Iodine is also necessary for maintaining connective tissue in the body that make up tendons and ligaments, holds tissues together, and is crucial for the development of a growing fetus. It is also important for the intellectual development of the child.

ABSORPTION HELPERS

The mineral selenium helps to convert iodine into the thyroid hormones; a lack of selenium levels in the body can reduce the effectiveness of this mineral in the diet. Vitamin A is also important for the proper functioning of the thyroid gland.

TOP SOURCES OF IODINE mcg/4oz. of food

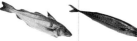

HADDOCK	SMOKED MACKEREL	MUSSELS	COD	LOBSTER
250mcg/4oz.	150mcg/4oz.	120mcg/4oz.	110mcg/4oz.	100mcg/4oz.

ABSORPTION INHIBITORS

Substances called glucosinolate progoitrin in cruciferous vegetables (especially in cabbage and turnips) prevent iodine absorption. Peanuts, cassava, and soy beans also block the action of iodine in the thyroid gland. The drug sulfonylurea, used in the treatment of adult onset or Type II diabetes, and cobalt and lithium antidepressants all decrease iodine uptake. Fluorine bromine and chlorine may affect the way iodine is used by the body.

TAKING IODINE SUPPLEMENTS

The adult RDA for iodine (150mcg) a day is found in one 4oz. serving of mackerel. Also available in multimineral and high-potency supplements in doses of 150mcg a day, the safe upper intake level is 700mcg a day in the short term and 500mcg in the long term. Iodine, taken as part of a multi-mineral with 100 percent of the RDA as a suitable way of self-supplementing; higher doses, should only be taken on the advice of a doctor. Kelp supplements are another optional source of iodine.

PRECAUTIONS

High intakes of iodine can lead to toxicity in the thyroid gland, resulting in swelling and possibly even cancer. Pregnant women should avoid high intakes of iodine, and acne sufferers may find the condition worsens when taking high levels of iodine supplements. Always check with your doctor before taking iodine supplements containing more than 100 percent of the RDA.

THERAPEUTIC USES

● SWOLLEN THYROID GLAND

A swollen thyroid gland, or goiter, is a symptom of iodine deficiency. If it is caused through a simple lack of iodine, modest amounts of supplements can help the swelling to reduce. Severe goiters require medical treatment with thyroxine or need to be surgically removed.

● PAINFUL BREASTS

Women suffering with benign swelling and lumpiness of the breasts have shown improvement in both the associated pain and formation of benign cysts when iodine intakes are increased.

● BREAST CANCER

Low intakes of iodine appear to be related to precancerous lesions in the breast tissue that are corrected when iodine intakes are restored to normal levels.

● WEIGHT PROBLEMS

Taking 100 percent of the RDA of iodine may help to improve the action of a sluggish thyroid gland and may also help to improve weight problems.

WHY TAKE THIS SUPPLEMENT?

Diets poor in diary food and seafood may be in short supply of iodine. Regularly eating large amounts of raw cabbage may also put a strain on iodine levels. Signs of low iodine levels include:

- ○ TIREDNESS
- ○ COLD HANDS AND FEET
- ○ POOR CONCENTRATION
- ○ FAILING MEMORY
- ○ MUSCLE WEAKNESS
- ○ BREAST PAIN
- ○ SUDDEN OR UNEXPLAINED BREAST PAIN
- ○ ENLARGED THYROID GLAND IN NECK

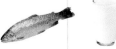

CANNED SALMON
59mcg/4oz.

HERRING
29mcg/4oz.

SHRIMP
28mcg/4oz.

STEAMED BROWN TROUT
16mcg/4oz.

MILK
15mcg/4oz.

POTASSIUM

Helps to lower raised blood pressure

Relieves muscle cramps ✦ Reduces the risk of stroke

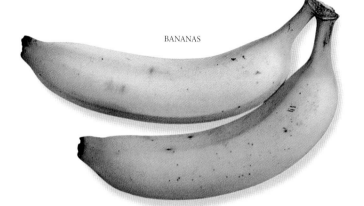

BANANAS

CHEMICAL NAMES

- POTASSIUM GLUCONATE
- POTASSIUM SULFATE
- POTASSIUM CHLORIDE
- POTASSIUM OXIDE
- POTASSIUM CARBONATE
- POTASSIUM GLUCONATE
- POTASSIUM CITRATE
- POTASSIUM FUMERATE

PREPARATIONS

- TABLETS
- POWDER
- CAPSULES

RDA FOR ADULTS

- NO RDA ESTABLISHED

HOW IT WORKS

Potassium is crucial for the smooth functioning of all muscles and nerves in the body. It also helps maintain the fluid levels in the body at the correct balance, and ensures that the correct balance of acid to alkaline is maintained. Much potassium in the body is located inside cells and is balanced by sodium, which stays outside these cells. One of its other important roles is to help prevent calcium being lost in the urine.

ABSORPTION HELPERS

Potassium is found in many fruits and vegetables, from which it is generally well-absorbed by the body.

ABSORPTION INHIBITORS

Too much sodium (pp.74 –75) from salt, processed foods, and excess alcohol can affect levels of potassium. Diuretic drugs, taken to reduce water retention, and cortico-steroid drugs, taken to reduce inflammation, can also disturb the balance of potassium in the body.

TOP SOURCES OF POTASSIUM mg/4oz. of food

TOMATO PUREE	SPINACH	PARSNIP	RADISH	WATERCRESS
1,150mg/4oz.	500mg/4oz.	450mg/4oz.	240mg/4oz.	230mg/4oz.

TAKING POTASSIUM SUPPLEMENTS

Although there is no RDA for potassium, the reference nutrient intake is set at 3,500mg a day, which is equivalent to eating two bananas, a serving of honeydew melon, eight apricots, two oranges, or a red pepper. Optimum nutritionists suggest intakes of 200mg a day for adults; daily therapeutic levels are set at 3,500mg. Potassium supplements should **always** be taken on the advice of a doctor. Potassium chloride, brewer's yeast, and potassium gluconate appear to be the most effective supplements.

PRECAUTIONS

Daily intakes of more than 17,600mg (17.6g) of potassium supplements may lead to toxicity. People with diabetes in particular should avoid taking potassium supplements unless they are prescribed by a doctor. It should also be understood that supplementing your diet with potassium may increase the loss of magnesium from the body, an important mineral necessary for maintaining strong bones and teeth.

THERAPEUTIC USES

● CONGESTIVE HEART FAILURE

Low levels of potassium are common in patients with congestive heart failure (where the heart is unable to pump enough blood around the body). The irregular heart rhythms that can result may be reduced by increasing intakes of potassium.

● KIDNEY STONES

Eating a potassium-rich diet can help to reverse high levels of calcium lost in the urine, which, if not corrected, can increase the risk of kidney stones.

● REDUCED RISK OF STROKE

Improved potassium intakes in the diet have been associated with a reduction in the risk of death from strokes.

● LOWERING HIGH BLOOD PRESSURE

High blood pressure has been linked to low levels of potassium in the diet. Potassium supplements work both for those whose blood pressure is raised through the use of diuretics, and for people with other causes of raised blood pressure.

● MUSCLE CRAMPS AND LOW POTASSIUM

Potassium chloride supplements may help those people who regularly experience muscle cramps. These cramps are caused either by low dietary intakes of potassium, or as a result of increased losses of the mineral from the body.

WHY TAKE THIS SUPPLEMENT?

A low dietary intake of potassium is unlikely; the mineral is widely distributed in foods – although elderly people on a limited diet containing few vegetables and fruit may be at risk of low intakes. However, losses can be great in those suffering prolonged cases of vomiting, diarrhea, or sweating, who experience blood loss, or who regularly take diuretics or laxatives. Other signs of low potassium levels in the body include:

❍ MUSCLE WEAKNESS
❍ DISORIENTATION
❍ IRRITABILITY
❍ CONFUSION
❍ DEPRESSION

PASSION FRUIT
200mg/4oz.

PAPAYA
200mg/4oz.

RED PEPPER
160mg/4oz.

PEACH
160mg/4oz.

RED WINE
130mg/4oz.

MAGNESIUM

May help reduce complications with diabetes ❖ May lower risk of heart disease ❖ Relieves premenstrual headaches

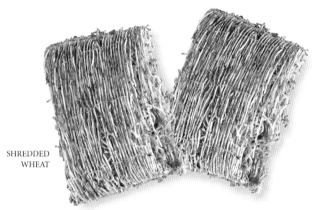

SHREDDED
WHEAT

CHEMICAL NAMES

- MAGNESIUM
  CARBONATE
- MAGNESIUM
  GLUCONATE
- MAGNESIUM OXIDE
- MAGNESIUM SULFATE

PREPARATIONS

- TABLETS
- CAPSULES
- POWDER
- DOLOMITE

RDA FOR ADULTS

- 350MG

HOW IT WORKS

Magnesium is stored in all body tissues and is needed for the growth and maintenance of strong bones and teeth. The mineral also plays an important role in helping muscles to relax and is necessary for a healthy heart and nervous system. Involved in the formation and action of over 300 different enzyme reactions, magnesium affects many body systems and helps in the release of energy from food and the protection of cell walls.

ABSORPTION HELPERS

Protein foods such as meat, chicken, fish, and eggs help magnesium absorption along with steady intakes of calcium. The minerals phosphorus and zinc, plus vitamins B1, B6, C, and D, are also thought to help improve magnesium absorption.

ABSORPTION INHIBITORS

Large amounts of calcium reduce the body's ability to absorb magnesium. This mineral binds to substances called "oxalates,"

TOP SOURCES OF MAGNESIUM mg/4oz. of food

COCOA POWDER	SUNFLOWER SEEDS	PUMPKIN SEEDS	ALL-BRAN	MIXED NUTS
520mg/4oz.	390mg/4oz.	270mg/4oz.	210mg/4oz.	200mg/4oz.

found in spinach and rhubarb as well as phytate in wheat bran. The long-term use of diuretics is also known to reduce body levels of magnesium.

TAKING MAGNESIUM SUPPLEMENTS

The RDA for magnesium (350mg) is found in one pint of milk, a serving of cod with spinach, a handful of peanuts, and four slices of bread. Take supplements on medical advice only. The safe upper level of intake is 300mg for long-term usage and 400mg for short-term usage. Optimum nutritionists set intakes at 375-500mg a day for adults and 400-800mg for therapeutic uses. Magnesium citrate is the form most easily absorbed by the body.

PRECAUTIONS

Excessive intakes are linked to paralysis, nausea, and depression. Daily doses of 3,000-5,000mg can be fatal.

THERAPEUTIC USES

● **DIABETES**
A deficiency of magnesium can occur in people with diabetes, and is associated with immediate and long-term complications – heart disease, kidney problems, and nerve damage. Essential for the transportation of glucose, magnesium is also important in the release of the hormone insulin, which helps to control blood sugar levels. Magnesium supplements may also benefit non-diabetics who experience symptoms of blood sugar lows, such as feeling light-headed or faint.

● **HEART ATTACKS**
Magnesium deficiency is associated with increased risk of heart disease and sudden cardiac death. Supplements may reduce the risk of irregular heartbeats after a heart attack.

● **HEART DISEASE**
Magnesium may help to reduce total cholesterol, raise "good" HDL cholesterol and stop blood from clotting, so limiting the risk of atherosclerosis and heart disease.

● **PAINFUL PERIODS**
Women who experience painful periods may find relief from back and lower stomach pain by taking magnesium. The effect may be enhanced if taken with vitamin B6.

● **PREMENSTRUAL HEADACHES**
Premenstrual headaches may be associated with low blood levels of magnesium. Intakes of 100–200mg daily may help.

WHY TAKE THIS SUPPLEMENT?

Supplements of magnesium are usually only given on the advice of a doctor, for example, after prolonged vomiting and diarrhea, high alcohol intakes, or those with kidney disease. However, women who suffer with symptoms of premenstrual syndrome and those concerned about an increased risk of osteoporosis may also benefit. Signs of low magnesium intakes include:

○ WEAKNESS
○ RAPID OR IRREGU–LAR HEARTBEAT
○ MUSCLE CRAMPS
○ LOSS OF APPETITE
○ NAUSEA
○ FATIGUE
○ INSOMNIA
○ VOMITING
○ ANOREXIA
○ PERSONALITY CHANGES

PEANUT BUTTER
180mg/4oz.

SHREDDED WHEAT
130mg/4oz.

RYE CRACKERS
100mg/4oz.

PLAIN POPCORN
81mg/4oz.

WHOLEWHEAT BISCUITS
75mg/4oz.

MANGANESE

Helps control blood sugar levels ❖ Reduces epileptic seizures

Improves bone strength ❖ May help in wound healing

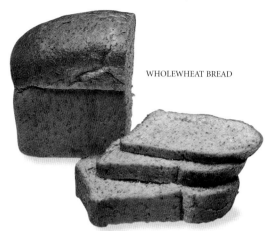

WHOLEWHEAT BREAD

CHEMICAL NAMES

- MANGANESE SULFATE
- MANGANESE GLUCONATE
- MANGANESE CITRATE
- (MANGANESE AMINO ACID CHELATE)

PREPARATIONS

- MANGANESE IS MAINLY FOUND AS PART OF MULTIVITAMIN AND MINERAL PREPARATIONS

RDA FOR ADULTS

- 2.5–5MG

HOW IT WORKS

Manganese is needed for certain enzymes to be activated to begin to work in the body. It is also crucial for the formation of other enzymes, including one called "superoxide dismutase," which breaks down potentially damaging free radicals capable of sparking heart disease and certain cancers. It is also needed to enable the body to make use of protein foods in the diet, and for the formation of sex hormones. Manganese is known to maintain the health of nerves and help lubricate joints, promote good bone structure, and aid the production of thyroid hormones, which control the speed of the body's metabolism. It is also thought to be involved in the balancing of blood sugar levels.

ABSORPTION HELPERS

Vitamin C, along with zinc and vitamins B1, E, and K, may help improve the absorption of manganese by the body.

TOP SOURCES OF MANGANESE mcg/4oz. of food

MACADAMIA NUTS	FILBERTS	PECANS	DESSICATED COCONUT	ALMONDS
5.5mcg/4oz.	4.9mcg/4oz.	4.6mcg/100g	1.8mcg/100g	1.7mcg/100g

Unusually, manganese absorption levels increase when iron intakes are low; and conversely, when iron intakes improve, the absorption levels of manganese decrease.

ABSORPTION INHIBITORS

Large intakes of calcium and phosphorus reduce levels of absorption, while antibiotics and too much alcohol and refined food can deplete body stores.

TAKING SUPPLEMENTS

While the RDA is 2.5–5mg, it is suggested that intakes should at least be above 1.4mg a day, an amount that can be found in three slices of wholewheat bread. Optimum nutritionists suggest intakes of 5mg daily, with therapeutic intakes ranging from 2.5mg to 15mg daily. The three most absorbable forms of manganese are: amino acid chelates, manganese gluconate, and manganese citrate.

PRECAUTIONS

Any excess manganese remains unabsorbed by the body, making this mineral one of the least toxic of all minerals found in the diet.

THERAPEUTIC USES

● IMPROVED BLOOD SUGAR LEVELS IN DIABETES

People with diabetes who have low levels of manganese have been shown to improve their responses to sugar in the blood when supplements are taken on a daily basis.

● EPILEPTIC SEIZURES

When manganese levels are low in people with epilepsy, supplements have been shown to help in the control of both major and minor seizures.

● IMPROVED IMMUNE SYSTEM

The immune systems of people who suffer from depression often have low resistance to infection. Manganese supplements seem to help strengthen the immune system.

● BONE STRENGTH

A lack of manganese, which is needed for good bone formation, has been found in women with reduced bone density – putting bones at greater risk of fracturing. Improving dietary intakes of manganese may strengthen bones and lower the risk of osteoporosis.

● IMPROVED WOUND HEALING

Good dietary intakes of manganese, needed for the formation of the wound-healing tissue collagen, may be important in all aspects of wound healing, especially following operations, when food intakes in patients can be poor.

WHY TAKE THIS SUPPLEMENT?

A lack of manganese is most unusual in normal mixed diets, and a specific supplement is considered unnecessary. However, optimum nutritionists suggest that those suffering from recurrent dizziness, or who are absent-minded, have memory problems, or eat a lot of dairy foods may benefit from a modest manganese supplement. Signs that manganese intakes may be low include:

○ JOINT PAIN
○ SKIN RASH
○ POOR MEMORY
○ MUSCLE TWITCHES
○ DIZZINESS
○ POOR BALANCE

CASHEW NUTS
1.7mcg/100g

SOYBEANS
0.9mcg/100g

BOILED BROWN RICE
0.9mcg/100g

GARBANZA BEANS
0.8mcg/100g

TEA
0.14mcg/100g

MOLYBDENUM

May reduce allergic symptoms

YELLOW SPLIT PEAS

ADUKI BEANS

BROWN LENTILS

CHEMICAL NAMES

- MOLYBDENUM

PREPARATIONS

- FOUND IN MULTIMINERAL PREPARATIONS

RDA FOR ADULTS

- 75–250MCG

HOW IT WORKS

Molybdenum is involved in the functioning of several important enzymes that help the body to make use of the energy from fat and carbohydrate in food, for example. The mineral is also important in allowing the body to make use of iron, and for keeping nerves healthy and sustaining good mental alertness. Molybdenum is also needed for maintaining male fertility and potency; a lack of it in the diet is a potential cause of impotence in older men. Molybdenum deficiency may also increase susceptibility to tooth decay, and a low intake is associated with mouth and gum disorders.

ABSORPTION HELPERS

Molybdenum is efficiently absorbed by the body, even when dietary intakes are very low.

ABSORPTION INHIBITORS

Excess silicon, taken in supplement form, can

TOP SOURCES OF MOLYBDENUM (no figures available)

LIVER

YEAST

LENTILS

SPINACH

GREEN CABBAGE

reduce the amount of molybdenum in the body, as can very high intakes of protein from animal food sources such as meat and poultry. Silicon supplements will reduce the plasma concentration and uptake of molybdenum, while too much copper increases the rate of molybdenum loss from the body.

TAKING MOLYBDENUM SUPPLEMENTS

The adult RDA for molybdenum is 75 to 250mcg, and safe intakes are thought to range between 50 and 400mcg a day, with current intakes estimated to be 25mcg. Levels in multimineral supplements tend to range from 100mcg up to 300mcg. Optimum nutritionists suggest adult intakes of between 100–1000mcg per day.

PRECAUTIONS

High intakes of 10,000-15,000mcg (10-15mg) of molybdenum increases the excretion of copper and may also raise levels of uric acid. Excess uric acid tends to accumulate in the joints, which can result in the development of gout, a painful and debilitating condition that must be treated with prescribed drugs.

THERAPEUTIC USES

● ALLERGY

If allergy sufferers have a molybdenum deficiency, supplementation may be beneficial: injections of molybdenum in amounts ranging from 250mcg to 750mcg for three months have been shown to reduce wheezing and the need for people with asthma to use inhalers. Supplements of molybdenum should not be undertaken without medical supervision.

● ASTHMA

Molybdenum may occasionally be prescribed for people who suffer from asthma who have difficulty in accommodating sulfites, which are used as preservatives in food manufacturing.

● DETOXIFIES SULFITES

Molybdenum appears to help the body break down sulfites. Extra intakes may be useful for people on refined, processed diets that contain large intakes of sulfite-containing preservatives.

WHY TAKE THIS SUPPLEMENT?

It is unlikely that the general population require specific supplementation with molybdenum. Multimineral supplements supplying this nutrient may be useful, however, for those people who eat a diet rich in refined foods and low in good sources of molybdenum – such as cereals and vegetables. Supplements may also be useful for those people who eat cereals and vegetables that have been grown on molybdenum-depleted soils, and also in areas of soft water, which is low in this mineral.

There are no known deficiency symptoms for a lack of molybdenum in the diet.

WHOLEWHEAT BREAD

WHOLEWHEAT PASTA

BROWN RICE

KIDNEY

RED KIDNEY BEANS

SODIUM

Needed in rehydration treatments for prolonged diarrhea
and vomiting ● May help improve night muscle cramps

TABLE SALT

CHEMICAL NAMES

• SODIUM CHLORIDE

PREPARATIONS

• TABLETS

RDA FOR ADULTS

• 500MG

HOW IT WORKS

Of the 120mg of sodium found in the body, about one third is located in the skeleton and the remaining two thirds is present in the body's fluids, which wash around the outside of the cells, and also in nerves and muscles. Sodium is essential for maintaining the water balance of the body and for making sure this balance becomes neither too acidic or alkaline. The mineral is needed by cell walls so they can take in nutrients from the blood, and also to enable muscle contraction.

ABSORPTION HELPERS

The human body has little difficulty in absorbing sodium from food and drink, with 95 percent of sodium moving from the intestine into the blood.

ABSORPTION INHIBITORS

Excessive intakes of the mineral potassium *(see pp.66–67)* can result in depleted levels of sodium in the body.

TOP SOURCES OF SODIUM mg/100g of food

TABLE SALT	SALAMI	PICKLE	OAT CRACKERS	TOMATO KETCHUP
38,850mg/4oz.	1,850mg/4oz.	1,700mg/4oz.	1,230mg/4oz.	1,120mg/4oz.

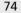

TAKING SODIUM SUPPLEMENTS

The RDA for sodium is 500mg, the recommended nutrient intake can easily be achieved by eating just one 1-oz slice of bacon. If supplements are considered to be necessary – through, for example, heat exhaustion, low blood pressure, or muscle cramps – they should only be taken under qualified medical supervision. Optimum nutritionists suggest intakes of 2,400mg daily.

PRECAUTIONS

High intakes of sodium can reduce the body's balance of potassium, lead to the retention of fluid, and, in large amounts, can be fatal. High intakes of sodium are also linked to raised blood pressure.

THERAPEUTIC USES

● **DIARRHEA**
Sodium levels in the body can drop as a result of prolonged vomiting and diarrhea. These levels are usually restored by taking specially formulated isotonic drinks or drips. Isotonic drinks contain the same balance of

sodium and potassium found in normal blood fluids and so quickly help to restore the appropriate levels required by the body.

● **RAPID FLUID REPLACEMENT**
Sodium is added to commercially available isotonic sports drinks to maximize the speed of water absorption and the rate of fluid rehydration in the body during and after exercising.

● **MUSCLE CRAMPS**
People with low levels of sodium who experience nighttime muscle cramps may benefit from modest increases of sodium chloride – better known as salt – to prevent this occurence.

● **EYE DROPS**
Sodium chloride is used to make solutions such as eye drops, saline, and artificial tears. The sodium helps make the artificial tears as similar as possible to the composition of human tears.

● **HEAT EXHAUSTION**
Exhaustion from strenuous physical activity or in high temperatures may require salt tablets and water to restore body fluid levels.

WHY TAKE THIS SUPPLEMENT?

The general population should not need supplements because sodium is so widely available from foods, especially refined and processed foods. Hard exercise in high temperatures causes sodium loss through sweating, which may need to be replaced by taking salt tablets. People with prolonged bouts of diarrhea or vomiting can also lose a lot of body fluids – which includes sodium – and may need to be replaced. When sodium levels are low in the body, dehydration can occur. The main signs of dehydration include:

❍ DIZZINESS
❍ LOW BLOOD PRESSURE
❍ MUSCLE CRAMPS
❍ DEHYDRATION
❍ NAUSEA AND VOMITING
❍ HEAT EXHAUSTION
❍ POOR CONCENTRATION
❍ HEADACHE
❍ LOSS OF APPETITE

CORNFLAKES
1,110mg/4oz.

POTATO CHIPS
1,070mg/4oz.

BRANFLAKES
1,000mg/4oz.

WHOLEWHEAT BREAD
550mg/4oz.

WHITE BREAD
520mg/4oz.

PHOSPHORUS

Essential for strong bones and teeth ✦ May improve
fracture healing ✦ May reduce tiredness in people with diabetes

COOKED
SHRIMP

CHEMICAL NAMES

- CALCIUM PHOSPHATE
- MONOSODIUM PHOSPHATE

PREPARATIONS

- TABLETS
- CAPSULES
- POWDER
- LIQUID

RDA FOR ADULTS

- 700MG

HOW IT WORKS

Phosphorus combines with calcium to form calcium phosphate, which plays a crucial role in making bones and teeth strong and rigid. While as much as 85 percent of the phosphorus in the body is stored in the skeleton, the remaining 15 percent has other vital roles. It is essential for the control and production of energy from carbohydrate and fat from food, and for the structure of both the genetic material known as DNA and phospholipids, which is found in every cell wall in the body.

ABSORPTION HELPERS

Vitamin D increases the absorption of phosphorus, and having the correct proportion of calcium to phosphorus also improves the absorption rate.

ABSORPTION INHIBITORS

Large amounts of calcium can reduce phosphorus levels in the body. The ideal ratio of calcium to phosphorus intakes is 2:1.

TOP SOURCES OF PHOSPHORUS mg/4oz. of food

CHEESE	LIVER	SHRIMP	CRAB	MUSSELS
490mg/4oz.	470mg/4oz.	350mg/4oz.	350mg/4oz.	330mg/4oz.

76

Excessive intakes of the minerals magnesium and aluminum can also impair phosphorus absorption. Long-term usage of antacids, which contain aluminum and magnesium hydroxide to help control acid indigestion, may also reduce phosphorus levels.

TAKING PHOSPHORUS SUPPLEMENTS

The adult RDA (700mg) is equivalent to having a pint of milk and a cheddar cheese sandwich. The safe upper level of intake is 1,500mg for short- and long-term use, which optimum nutritionists agree with. The best forms of supplements are calcium phosphate, and monosodium phosphate.

PRECAUTIONS

Cola drinks are rich in phosphoric acid. Large amounts may cause excessive phosphorous intakes, which may in turn affect calcium levels.

THERAPEUTIC USES

● **BONE DENSITY**
Recent evidence suggests that dietary phosphorus has an important role to play in the development of peak bone mass (PBM). Phosphate makes up roughly half the weight of bone and therefore must be present in the diet in adequate amounts to maintain the skeleton. Intakes of 1g of phosphorus a day may reduce the amount of time fractures take to heal and reduce mineral loss from immobile limbs.

● **HIGH ALCOHOL INTAKES**
People who consume high levels of alcohol often have low levels of blood phosphate, and so may be treated with phosphorus supplements. These supplements can also be useful in the treatment of withdrawal from alcohol.

● **DIABETES**
There is a small amount of evidence to suggest that reducing tiredness and improving the control of diabetes in insulin-dependent diabetics is possible by taking supplements.

● **KIDNEY STONES**
Taking orthophosphate supplements appears to lower the rate of kidney stone formation by helping to reduce urinary levels of calcium.

● **FRACTURE HEALING**
One gram of phosphorus per day has been used to reduce the healing time of ankle and femur fractures.

WHY TAKE THIS SUPPLEMENT?

People taking a long course of antacids or who drink large amounts of alcohol may need to take phosphorus supplements. People with Crohn's disease and poorly controlled diabetes may also benefit. In the general population deficiency is rare because it is so widely available in the diet. Signs of a lack of phosphorus include:

❍ LOW BONE DENSITY
❍ WEAKENED, SOFT BONES
❍ FAILURE TO GROW
❍ WEAKNESS
❍ TIREDNESS
❍ ANOREXIA
❍ TWITCHING
❍ MUSCLE SPASMS IN THE HANDS, FACE, AND FEET

LOBSTER
280mg/4oz.

SMOKED SALMON
250mg/4oz.

STEAK
170mg/4oz.

TURKEY
220mg/4oz.

NATURAL YOGURT
160mg/4oz.

SELENIUM

May reduce the risk of cancer ❖ May protect against heart disease ❖ Strengthens the immune system ❖ Helps acne

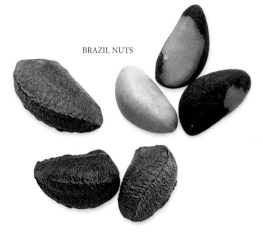

BRAZIL NUTS

CHEMICAL NAMES

- L-SELENOMETHIONINE
- SODIUM SELENITE

PREPARATIONS

- TABLETS
- CAPSULES

RDA FOR ADULTS

- 55–70MCG

HOW IT WORKS

Selenium works as part of an antioxidant system that helps to protect body cells from damage by free radicals, which may otherwise trigger heart disease and some cancers. Selenium in the body helps to bind with metals such as arsenic and mercury, which otherwise may be toxic and cause illness. Selenium is also involved in the production and maintenance of healthy sperm and the prostate gland in men.

ABSORPTION HELPERS

The presence of vitamins A, C, and E appear to help in the body's absorption of selenium.

ABSORPTION INHIBITORS

The availability of selenium depends on the nature of the food, its processing and preparation, and the health of the digestive tract's absorbent surfaces. Too much sulfur in the diet can reduce selenium absorption. Highly processed foods can be stripped of much

TOP SOURCES OF SELENIUM mcg/4oz. of food

BRAZIL NUTS	MIXED NUTS & RAISINS	FRESH TUNA	SHRIMP	SUNFLOWER SEEDS
1,530mcg/4oz.	170mcg/4oz.	57mcg/4oz.	49mcg/4oz.	49mcg/4oz.

of their original selenium content. Inorganic selenium should be taken separately from vitamin C, which may impair its absorption.

TAKING SELENIUM SUPPLEMENTS

The adult RDA for selenium nutrient intake is 55–70mcg daily, which can be obtained by eating four to five Brazil nuts. Optimum nutritionists recommend 100mcg per day. Selenium bound to protein and known as selenomethionine is considered one of the best forms of supplement.

PRECAUTIONS

Selenium can be toxic in doses of 3,200mcg (3.2mg) to 6,700mcg (6.7mg) daily, and can lead to dry, brittle hair and hair loss, and bad breath. It is advisable to not take more than 200mcg daily.

THERAPEUTIC USES

● **ACNE**
Selenium is needed in the formation of the enzyme glutathione. In a study on people with severe pustular acne and low glutathione peroxidase activity, when a daily

combination of 200mg of selenium and 10mg of vitamin E were taken, improvements could be seen within 6–12 weeks.

● **CANCER**
It has been shown that people who have diets rich in selenium have lower rates of cancer than those people who have poor intakes of this mineral in their diet. Studies are currently assessing whether taking selenium supplements actually helps to reduce the risk of various cancers, especially those of the lung, prostate gland, colon, and rectum.

● **IMMUNE SYSTEM STIMULANT**
Low selenium intakes seem to allow otherwise harmless viruses to become active. Selenium supplements appear to stimulate the immune system, which in turn helps protect the body from infections.

● **HEART HEALTH**
Too much "bad" LDL cholesterol can trigger heart disease and stroke. Selenium benefits the heart by helping reduce this fatty buildup that clogs artery walls, and reduce damage to artery walls by free radical attack.

WHY TAKE THIS SUPPLEMENT?

Those people with a family history of heart disease and cancer, or who follow a vegan, vegetarian, or weight-loss diet, the elderly, pregnant and nursing mothers, and smokers may benefit from a modest selenium supplement. Signs of a lack of selenium in the diet include:

○ LOW MALE FERTILITY
○ DANDRUFF
○ WEAK MUSCLES
○ FREQUENT INFECTIONS
○ PREMATURE SIGNS OF AGING
○ POOR PROSTATE HEALTH

BROILED FLOUNDER
45mcg/4oz.

WHOLEWHEAT BREAD
35mcg/4oz.

CASHEW NUTS
29mcg/4oz.

WALNUTS
19mcg/4oz.

WHITE RICE
4mcg/4oz.

SILICON

Potential anti-aging properties ✦ May improve fragile nails
and brittle hair ✦ May reduce the risk of heart disease

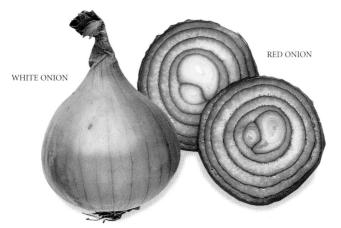

RED ONION

WHITE ONION

CHEMICAL NAMES

- SILICON
- SILICA
- SILICIC ACID

PREPARATIONS

- CAPSULES
- TABLETS
- HORSETAIL-CAPSULES
  AND TABLETS
- GEL

RDA

- HUMAN REQUIREMENTS
  FOR SILICON ARE NOT
  YET KNOWN.

HOW IT WORKS

The specific roles and requirement of silicon in the human diet are still under investigation. However, it is known that of all the body tissues, silicon levels are highest in the aorta (the main artery of the heart), the windpipe, lungs, and connective tissue. It is also found in bones. Silicon seems to give strength and firmness to these tissues, helping, for example, to keep the arteries in good condition. Silicon levels appear to decrease with age in the heart arteries, and with the development of atherosclerosis, suggesting that it may play a role in reducing the risk of heart disease. Silicon appears to be important in the early stages of new bone and tendon formation, which occurs throughout life and helps to keep these tissues in a good, healthy condition. It may also support and strengthen new hair and nail growth, and could counteract the effects of aluminum, which may

TOP SOURCES OF SILICON (no figures available)

WHEAT

MILO

OATS

BARLEY

RICE

give it a role in helping the prevention of Alzheimer's disease and osteoporosis.

ABSORPTION HELPERS

Most dietary silicon in the form of silica remains unabsorbed, in contrast to silicic acid, which is found in food and drink, and is well absorbed by the body. The minerals boron, calcium, magnesium, manganese, and potassium are thought to improve the body's ability to use silicic acid effectively.

ABSORPTION INHIBITORS

Too much molybdenum seems to reduce the required levels of silicon in the body's tissues.

TAKING SUPPLEMENTS

No RDA or reference nutrient intake level has been set for silicon, but it is estimated that people eat between 1.2g and 29g per day. Specific silicon supplements are now available, and intakes of 500mg (0.5g) three times a day are suggested by some clinical nutritionists.

PRECAUTIONS

Toxic effects are confined to the inhalation of silica as dust from coal, or glass

manufacture, sandblasting of rocks, and ceramics production that leads to lung damage.

THERAPEUTIC USES

Little scientific research has been carried out on the therapeutic value of silicon supplements. A few studies, together with anecdotal evidence and theoretical uses, suggest it may be useful for:

● HEART DISEASE
Increasing silicon intakes with age may improve the elasticity of artery walls and help reduce the risk of heart disease in later life.

● BRITTLE HAIR AND HAIR LOSS
Extra silicon in the diet in the form of 10ml of silicic acid gel daily for 90 days has been shown to improve fragile hair and brittle nails. It is also thought to help reduce hair loss.

● SMOOTH SKIN
Through its ability to strengthen connective tissue such as collagen (the underlying structure that holds skin in place), good dietary intakes of silicon may help to slow down the development of wrinkles.

● PREMATURE SKIN AGING
In tests conducted over 90 days, treatment with 10ml of silicic acid in gel form and a twice-daily application of silicic acid gel directly on the skin for ten minutes at a time showed an improved elasticity of the skin and a reduced thickening associated with aging.

● STOMACH SETTLING
Silicic acid taken in gel form may help improve digestion. By forming a coat over the stomach wall, the silicic acid is thought to absorb toxins and irritants from food, which are then passed out of the body to reduce abdominal discomfort.

WHY TAKE THIS SUPPLEMENT?

No clear deficiency symptoms are associated with silicon, but signs that intakes may need to be improved include:
○ PEELING NAILS
○ WHITE SPOTS ON NAILS
○ OSTEOPOROSIS
○ WRINKLED SKIN
○ WEAK, BRITTLE HAIR

ONIONS

BEETS

ALFALFA

HARD WATER

HORSETAIL HERB

SULFUR

Promotes healthy joints, strong hair and nails

Provides allergy relief ◆ Helpful for detoxification

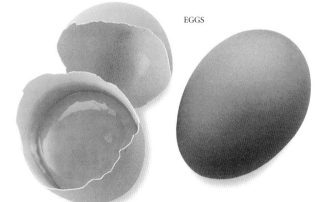

EGGS

CHEMICAL NAMES

- SULFUR

PREPARATIONS

- METHYLSULFONYL-
  METHONE (MSM)

RDA FOR ADULTS

- NO RDA HAS BEEN
  ESTABLISHED

HOW IT WORKS

Sulfur is vital for the production of keratin, a protein involved in the healthy structure of the hair and skin. An essential mineral that is present in all body cells, it is needed for the correct formation of the cartilage between bones, for the tendons which attach muscles to bones, and in the structure of bones themselves. Sulfur is also needed for the production of the hormone insulin, which keeps blood sugar levels balanced, and for heparin, which is involved in blood-clotting processes. Sulfur is also involved in creating and maintaining a healthy reproductive system and in keeping the lining of both arteries and veins intact. In addition, this mineral plays a part in the detoxification of alcohol, any cyanide consumed through its presence in foods, inhaled pollutants in the atmosphere, and tobacco smoke. This detoxification occurs

TOP SOURCES OF SULFUR (no figures available)

EGGS

LENTILS

PORK

BEEF

CHICKEN

by the particular toxic compound binding with sulfur, and then both elements are passed out of the body in the urine.

ABSORPTION HELPERS

Sulfur is present in certain amino acids, which are a particularly well-absorbed source of this mineral. Vitamin E helps keep the sulfur from amino acids intact in the body, making them available for uptake and use by the relevant body cells.

ABSORPTION INHIBITORS

Excess levels of copper in the diet can attach to the mineral, making it difficult to absorb.

TAKING SULFUR SUPPLEMENTS

Sulfur is mainly added to creams and ointments rather than to supplements. The former can be very effective in treating a variety of skin problems. One of the chemical forms of sulfur, sulfate, can be found in chondroitin supplements.

PRECAUTIONS

There is no known toxicity from the sulfur that is consumed as part of protein, although

sulfate compounds such as sodium sulfate – a food additive that acts as a dilutant – potassium sulfate, which is used as an alternative to salt, and calcium and magnesium sulfate, which are added increase the firm texture of foods, are not advisable.

THERAPEUTIC USES

● **JOINT HEALTH**
Chondroitin, found in the gristle around bone joints in the body, helps to draw fluid to cells in the joint, which acts as a lubricant to allow the bones to glide smoothly. It also works with glucosamine to replenish collagen and other building blocks of cartilage. Several studies suggest that people with arthritis who are given chondroitin sulfate supplements subsequently experience both pain relief and better joint movement, which could be due to the production of new cartilage.

● **DETOXIFICATION**
Adequate levels of sulfur in the human diet may help the body to detoxify itself of alcohol, traces of environmental pollutants, and other substances such as cyanide.

● **STRONG HAIR AND NAILS**
Good intakes of sulfur help to promote the growth and maintenance of strong, healthy hair and nails.

● **ARTHRITIC PAIN RELIEF**
Trials have been conducted with intravenous sulfur used as a supplement, which has shown a reduction in pain by sufferers of osteoarthritis and rheumatoid arthritis.

● **ALLERGY RELIEF**
Methylsulfonlymethane (MSM) is an organic sulfur supplement that appears to relieve allergic symptoms when two 1,000mg tablets are combined with vitamin C and bioflanonoids.

WHY TAKE THIS SUPPLEMENT?

There is no evidence that extra amounts of sulfur are needed in supplement form by people who have a balanced diet with adequate amounts of protein. However, supplements that contain chondroitin sulfates have been developed for people with arthritis.

TURKEY

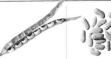

RED KIDNEY BEANS

BLACK-EYED PEAS

CANNELLINI BEANS

PEAS

ZINC

May help improve acne ✦ Helps reduce the symptoms of a large prostate gland ✦ May improve wound healing

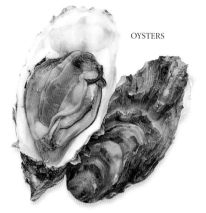

OYSTERS

CHEMICAL NAMES

- ZINC PICOLINATE
- ZINC GLUCONATE
- ZINC ASPARTATE

PREPARATIONS

- TABLETS
- CAPSULES
- LOZENGES

RDA FOR ADULTS

- 12–15MG

HOW IT WORKS

Approximately 1.5g–2.5g of zinc in the body is distributed in organs, tissues, fluids, and secretions, and is crucial for the proper action of over 70 enzymes involved in a wide range of activities. Zinc plays a vital role in the growth of children and is especially important for the production of healthy sperm. It is also necessary for the immune system and for the healing of wounds. It helps to detoxify harmful metals such as cadmium and lead, and is involved in keeping sight, smell, and taste in good working order. It is also vital for the release of insulin.

ABSORPTION HELPERS

Adequate amounts of protein in the diet can help to improve zinc levels in the body.

ABSORPTION INHIBITORS

Fiber in cereals and phytates in pulses and spinach can reduce zinc absorption, as can too much phosphorus. The

TOP SOURCES OF ZINC mg/4oz. of food

OYSTERS	WHEATGERM	CALVES' LIVER	PUMPKIN SEEDS	CANNED CORNED BEEF
59.2mg/4oz.	17mg/4oz.	7.8mg/4oz.	6.6mg/4oz.	5.6mg/4oz.

84

oral contraceptive pill can lower levels of zinc, while the drug tetracycline, prescribed for acne and infections, interferes with the absorption of zinc.

TAKING ZINC SUPPLEMENTS

The RDA for zinc (12–15mg) can be obtained from an 8-oz. steak. Optimum nutritionists suggest intakes of 15-20mg a day, rising to 50mg for therapeutic uses. The suggested safe upper level of supplements is 15mg for long-term usage and 50mg for short-term usage. The body seems to tolerate zinc supplements in the form of zinc gluconate with ease. All types of zinc should be taken with food to avoid any nausea.

PRECAUTIONS

Daily intakes of 50-300mg of zinc over long periods of time can interfere with the absorption of iron and copper, leading to deficiencies in both. Symptoms such as nausea, vomiting, abdominal pain, and fever may occur after intakes of 2000mg (2g) or more. Anyone suffering from liver or intestinal damage should consult a doctor before taking supplements.

THERAPEUTIC USES

● ACNE
Studies have shown that some people who suffer from acne can have reduced levels of zinc. Daily supplements of 200mg of zinc gluconate, which is equivalent to 30mg of pure zinc, is linked to improvements in inflammation.

● PROSTATE AND SPERM HEALTH
Symptoms of benign prostatic hyperplasia, such as a frequent need to pass urine, may be improved by taking 30mg of zinc daily. Good intakes of zinc may also improve male fertility since it is needed for damping down sperm activity until in the female tract.

● ECZEMA
People with eczema may have lowered levels of blood zinc. Modest daily supplements may help to significantly improve the condition in six weeks.

● WOUND HEALING
Wounds that take longer to heal than usual, often from a lack of zinc in the diet, may be improved by taking modest daily zinc supplements.

WHY TAKE THIS SUPPLEMENT?

People with acne, eczema, those who have recently undergone surgery or been badly burned, people over 55, men with a noncancerous swelling of the prostrate gland (benign prostatic hyperplasia), those suffering from a cold, and anyone on a restricted diet may benefit from zinc supplements. Signs of zinc deficiency can also include:

○ POOR GROWTH IN CHILDHOOD
○ DELAYED PUBERTY
○ DRY, ROUGH SKIN
○ ECZEMA
○ REPEATED AND FREQUENT INFECTIONS
○ LOSS OF APPETITE
○ LOSS OF TASTE
○ DIARRHEA
○ IMPAIRED SENSE OF SMELL AND SIGHT
○ POOR HEALING OF WOUNDS
○ POOR CONCENTRATION
○ SLOW GROWTH OF NAILS AND HAIR

ROAST BEEF
5.5mg/4oz.

LEAN ROAST LAMB
5.3mg/4oz.

CANNED CRAB
5.0mg/4oz.

PORK LOIN
3.5mg/4oz.

SARDINES IN OIL
3.0mg/4oz.

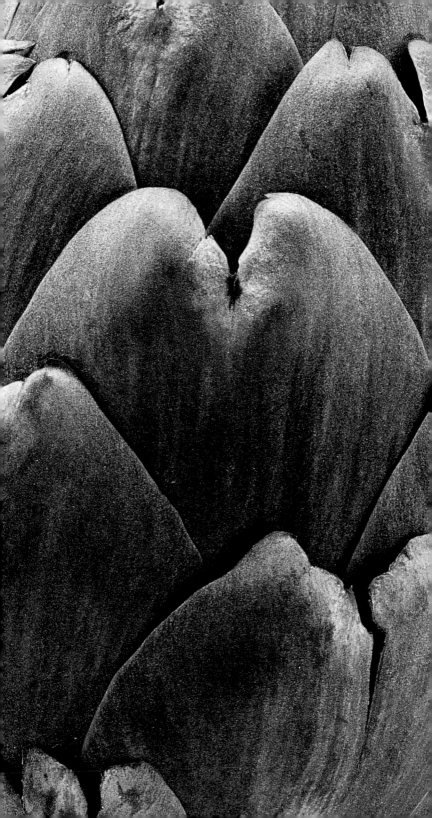

Other Supplements

Herbal remedies are not new, but the scientific
and medical world's interest in them is, as
research continues to prove the healing powers
of herbs. New plant nutrients are being found,
and their potential health benefits investigated.

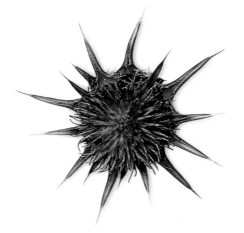

ARTICHOKE

May help to reduce the risk of heart disease ✛ Can help protect the liver from disease ✛ Relieves indigestion

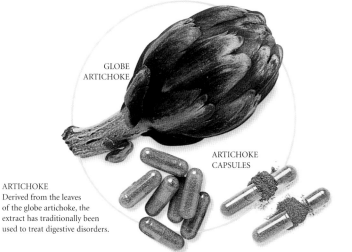

GLOBE
ARTICHOKE

ARTICHOKE
CAPSULES

ARTICHOKE
Derived from the leaves
of the globe artichoke, the
extract has traditionally been
used to treat digestive disorders.

PREPARATIONS

• TINCTURES
• CAPSULES

RECOMMENDED DAILY ADULT INTAKES

• 1–2 X 320MG CAPSULES

PRECAUTIONS

THOSE PEOPLE WHO ARE
SENSITIVE TO ARTICHOKES
IN THEIR DIET MAY
DEVELOP AN ALLERGIC
REACTION AND SHOULD
AVOID SUPPLEMENTS, AS
SHOULD PREGNANT AND
BREASTFEEDING WOMEN.

HOW IT WORKS

The active ingredients in artichoke extract, which are responsible for its actions in the body, include the cynaroside substances aglycone and luteolin, and the antioxidants caffeic acid, cynarin, and cholorgenic acid.

These substances all appear to protect liver cells from damage and stimulate the production of bile acid, which is released from the gall bladder into the digestive tract to help in the breakdown of fats and fat digestion. These active ingredients also appear to play a role in reducing the production of "bad" LDL cholesterol.

THERAPEUTIC USES

● **HEART DISEASE**
By reducing "bad" LDL cholesterol production, artichoke extracts may reduce atherosclerosis and the risk of heart disease.

● **INDIGESTION**
The stimulating effects artichoke extract has on the liver and gallbladder suggest that the body can deal better with both fat and alcohol as a result of taking artichoke supplements, which also may relieve indigestion after a large meal.

● **LIVER HEALTH**
Artichoke's antioxidant properties appear to help protect the liver from the risk of disease.

BIOFLAVONOIDS

Help treat asthma • Speed up healing of canker sores and bleeding gums • Slow down the skin's aging process

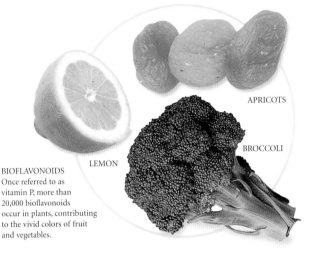

APRICOTS

BROCCOLI

LEMON

BIOFLAVONOIDS
Once referred to as vitamin P, more than 20,000 bioflavonoids occur in plants, contributing to the vivid colors of fruit and vegetables.

PREPARATIONS

- TABLETS
- CAPSULES

RECOMMENDED DAILY ADULT INTAKES

- INTAKES SEEM TO BE SAFE AT LEVELS OF 1,000MG

PRECAUTIONS

BIOFLAVONOIDS ARE NATURALLY OCCURRING SUBSTANCES THAT APPEAR TO HAVE VIRTUALLY NO TOXICITY.

HOW THEY WORK

Thousands of bioflavonoids occur in plants. Once in the body, they help prevent vitamin C from being destroyed and enhance the transportation of nutrients across blood vessels to body cells. Some bioflavonoids are powerful antioxidants that may protect the body from cancer, while others seem to have anti-inflammatory and anti-infection properties. Used in pharmacological doses, they may block certain enzymes and prevent cataracts.

THERAPEUTIC USES

● ASTHMA
Synthetic bioflavonoids, mimicking the anti-inflammatory properties of the natural substance, are used in asthma medications.

● CANKER SORES
When 100mg bioflavonoid supplements are taken with 100mg of vitamin C, it has been shown that the healing time of canker sores may reduce by a few days.

● BLEEDING GUMS
The bioflavonoid rutin helps strengthen tiny blood vessels and has been used to treat bleeding gums and varicose veins when taken with vitamin C.

● ANTI-AGING EFFECTS
Diets rich in bioflavonoids may improve the flexibility of skin and help slow down its aging process.

BLACK COHOSH

Provides effective pain relief ⬦ Can alleviate respiratory problems ⬦ Provides relief from rheumatoid arthritis

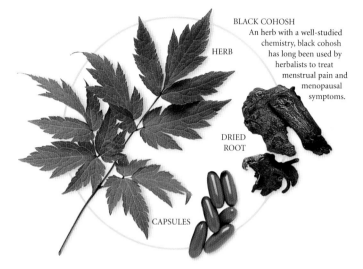

BLACK COHOSH
An herb with a well-studied chemistry, black cohosh has long been used by herbalists to treat menstrual pain and menopausal symptoms.

HERB

DRIED ROOT

CAPSULES

PREPARATIONS

- CAPSULES
- TABLETS
- TINCTURE

RECOMMENDED DAILY ADULT INTAKES

- 10-30 DROPS TINCTURE DAILY IN WATER OR TEA
- A 40MG CAPSULE OR TABLET ONCE DAILY

PRECAUTIONS

DO NOT USE DURING PREGNANCY OR WHEN BREASTFEEDING. USE IN SMALL AMOUNTS UNDER MEDICAL SUPERVISION JUST BEFORE GIVING BIRTH TO RELIEVE CONTRACTIONS. AVOID TAKING FOR PERIODS OF MORE THAN 6 MONTHS.

HOW IT WORKS

Shown to relieve menopausal symptoms by inhibiting the action of certain hormones, black cohosh is also stated to have antirheumatic, sedative, and antispasmodic properties. Salicylic acid *(see also p.125)* is among one of black cohosh's pain-relieving constituents.

THERAPEUTIC USES

● PAIN RELIEF

Black cohosh is an effective remedy for pain, especially for period pains, premenstrual syndrome, and during childbirth. Its antispasmodic action helps to ease and regulate uterine contractions.

● MENOPAUSE

The herb is used to treat menopausal symptoms, especially irritability, hot flashes, sleeplessness, and mild depression.

● ARTHRITIS

Black cohosh may alleviate the symptoms of sciatica and rheumatoid arthritis.

● RESPIRATORY PROBLEMS

Herbalists use black cohosh to treat stubborn coughs in asthma, whooping cough, and bronchitis.

● TINNITUS AND HEADACHES

Black cohosh is used by herbalists to treat tinnitus, a distressing ringing or buzzing in the ears.

CAROTENOIDS

May prevent age-related blindness ◦ May reduce the risk
of heart disease ◦ May reduce the risk of cancers

CAROTENOIDS
Carotenoids are the
pigments that give
vegetables and fruit their
rich colors, from the
luminous yellow of
lemons to the deep
red of tomatoes.

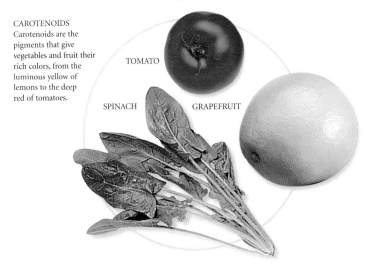

TOMATO

SPINACH   GRAPEFRUIT

PREPARATIONS

• CAPSULES
• TABLETS

RECOMMENDED DAILY ADULT INTAKES

• 6–20MG LUTEIN DAILY
• 3–6MG MIXED CAROTENOIDS
• 6–10MG LYCOPENE WITH MEALS
• 30–130MG ZEAXANTHIN

PRECAUTIONS

HIGH DOSES OF BETA-
CAROTENE SUPPLEMENTS
MAY INCREASE THE RISK
OF LUNG CANCER IN
HEAVY SMOKERS.

HOW IT WORKS

Carotenoids have anti-
oxidant properties and are
able to deactivate excess
free radicals that might
otherwise lead to an
increased risk of cancers
and heart disease.
Carotenoid compounds
include alpha- and beta-
carotene, cryptoxanthin,
lycopene, and zeaxanthin.
Beta-carotene in carrots
helps the eyes adapt to
dim light and can be
converted into vitamin A
if stores are low, while the
yellow lutein in corn and
spinach may help to
reduce the risk of macular
degeneration. Carotenoids
may also help to protect
the skin from UV
radiation damage.

THERAPEUTIC USES

● **BLINDNESS**
Lutein and zeaxanthin may
help prevent age-related
macular degeneration.

● **CANCER PREVENTION**
Diets rich in green,
yellow, and orange
vegetables may reduce the
risk of cancer, especially
of the lung and stomach.

● **HEART DISEASE**
Rates of heart disease have
been found to be lower in
countries where regular
intakes of tomatoes and
tomato-based products
are consumed.

● **CERVICAL CANCER**
Cryptoxanthin in peaches,
oranges, and papaya may
protect against this cancer.

CHITOSAN

Might aid weight loss

May help to lower total blood cholesterol

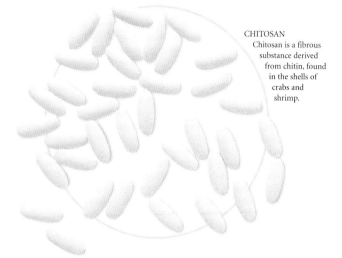

CHITOSAN
Chitosan is a fibrous substance derived from chitin, found in the shells of crabs and shrimp.

PREPARATIONS

- CAPSULES
- POWDER
- TABLETS
- LIQUID

RECOMMENDED DAILY ADULT INTAKES

- UP TO 2,000MG

PRECAUTIONS

CHITOSAN IS NOT SUITABLE FOR PEOPLE WITH AN ALLERGY TO SHELLFISH AND SHOULD NOT BE USED BY CHILDREN OR PREGNANT OR BREASTFEEDING WOMEN. IT MUST BE TAKEN WITH WATER. LONG-TERM USE MAY REDUCE ABSORPTION OF VITAMINS A, D, AND E.

HOW IT WORKS

In laboratory studies chitosan has been shown to bind up to six times its own weight of fat. It is suggested, but has never been proven, that this "fat-binding" effect also occurs in the human digestive tract. This has lead to the assumption that both the chitosan and the fat, which is attached, can pass out of the body in the stools so the fat calories are not actually absorbed by the body.

THERAPEUTIC USES

● **WEIGHT LOSS**
Although there is as yet no strong scientific proof to back up their views, manufacturers of chitosan supplements believe they can help reduce the absorption of fat and therefore fat calories, which can help lead to weight loss.

● **LOWERS CHOLESTEROL**
It has been suggested that chitosan can help to lower total blood cholesterol in conjunction with a healthy diet, and may even raise levels of "good" HDL cholesterol.

Co-ENZYME Q10

Benefits heart health ✦ Reduces inflammation of

gum disease ✦ May prevent senility and Alzheimer's disease

CO-ENZYME Q10
Co-enzyme Q10 is found
naturally in seafood, meats,
and whole grains, and
occurs throughout
the body.

PREPARATIONS

- CAPSULES
- GEL CAPSULES
- TABLETS

RECOMMENDED DAILY ADULT INTAKES

- 30–300MG

PRECAUTIONS

THOSE TAKING WARFARIN, A BLOOD-THINNING DRUG, SHOULD SEEK MEDICAL ADVICE BEFORE TAKING CO-ENZYME Q10.

HOW IT WORKS

Co-enzyme Q10, as its name suggests, is a substance needed by enzymes to assist them in their activities in the cells of the body, helping energy production. Levels of co-enzyme Q10 often decline with age.

Co-enzyme Q10 works specifically in the cells of nerves located in the heart and brain, and is particularly active in the liver, where it helps in the production of enzymes and hormones, and the breakdown of toxins. CoQ-10 (as it is often known) also has antioxidant functions, helping protect tissues from free radical damage, especially in the heart.

THERAPEUTIC USES

● **HEART HEALTH**
CoQ-10 strengthens the heart and, when taken under medical supervision, may help in conjunction with traditional treatments for congestive heart failure. It may also help lower blood pressure and reduce the risk of stroke and heart disease.

● **GUM DISEASE**
Taking 60mg of CoQ-10 a day may help reduce any inflammation associated with gum disease.

● **ANTI-AGING**
CoQ-10 appears to have the potential for use in treating and preventing symptoms of senility and Alzheimer's disease.

CLA

Can aid in fat loss ◈ May reduce the risk of heart disease ◈ May have anticancer effects

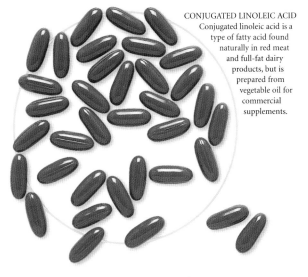

CONJUGATED LINOLEIC ACID
Conjugated linoleic acid is a type of fatty acid found naturally in red meat and full-fat dairy products, but is prepared from vegetable oil for commercial supplements.

PREPARATIONS

- CAPSULES
- POWDER

RECOMMENDED DAILY ADULT INTAKES

- TO MATCH DIETARY INTAKES FROM 30 YEARS AGO, WHICH HAVE FALLEN DUE TO A REDUCTION IN RED MEAT AND FULL-FAT DIARY FOODS, 3,000MG OR 3G OF CLA IS RECOMMENDED.

PRECAUTIONS

SOME FORMS OF CLA MAY CAUSE STOMACH IRRITATIONS. MICELLE VERSIONS ARE THE BEST TOLERATED.

HOW IT WORKS

Conjugated linoleic acid, or CLA, appears to help remove fat from fat cells and transport them to muscle tissue where it is burned as fuel. Laboratory research also suggests that CLA may be "cytotoxic" to breast and colon cancers, and may also protect against skin cancer. CLA also appears to reduce blood cholesterol and blood fats.

THERAPEUTIC USES

● FAT LOSS

Preliminary research in animals and humans suggests that CLA helps reduce body fat while maintaining muscle and bone tissue.

● CANCER PROTECTION

Early laboratory work reveals that CLA may reduce the risk of cancers of the breast, skin, colon, and rectum.

● HEART DISEASE

CLA may play a role in reducing the risk of heart disease by lowering LDL or "bad" cholesterol and blood fats.

● BONE STRENGTH

CLA may help to improve bone strength, which could help reduce the incidence of osteoporosis in later life.

DANDELION

Benefits liver ⊕ Effective in body detoxification
treatments ⊕ Can help relieve water retention

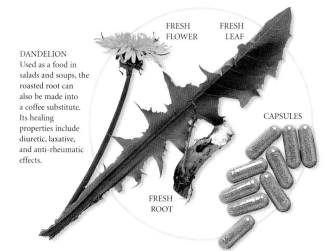

FRESH
FLOWER

FRESH
LEAF

DANDELION
Used as a food in
salads and soups, the
roasted root can
also be made into
a coffee substitute.
Its healing
properties include
diuretic, laxative,
and anti-rheumatic
effects.

CAPSULES

FRESH
ROOT

PREPARATIONS

- CAPSULES
- TABLETS
- LIQUID TINCTURE

RECOMMENDED DAILY ADULT INTAKES

- 1–3 CAPSULES
- 2–4 DROPS TINCTURE, 1-3 TIMES DAILY
- FRESH LEAVES IN A SALAD
- 1 CUP DANDELION TEA

PRECAUTIONS

DANDELION SUPPLEMENTS SHOULD BE AVOIDED BY ANYONE WITH AN INFLAMED GALL BLADDER OR BLOCKED BILE DUCT. THEY SHOULD ALSO BE AVOIDED WHILE TAKING DIURETIC MEDICINES.

HOW IT WORKS

Dandelion leaf extracts contain active constituents that appear to have a diuretic effect, increasing urination. This may help lower blood pressure and relieve water retention. Its rich source of potassium also helps improve the body's water balance. Bitter substances in extracts of dandelion root have a long history of helping treat liver and bile problems, which aid the digestive process.

THERAPEUTIC USES

● LIVER PROBLEMS
Dandelion may help in the treatment of liver problems such as cirrhosis, hepatitis, and liver toxicity.

● WATER RETENTION
Dandelion may help treat water retention and bloating, but supplements should not be taken without first obtaining medical advice.

● DETOXIFICATION
With its ability to improve liver and gall bladder activity, dandelion is often included in general dietary detoxification programs.

● INDIGESTION
By enhancing the action of the gall bladder and stimulating bile flow, dandelion extracts may help to improve fat digestion and relieve indigestion, bloating, gas, and constipation.

DEVIL'S CLAW

Can help relieve backache ◦ May relieve symptoms of arthritis ◦ Helps maintain healthy joints and ligaments

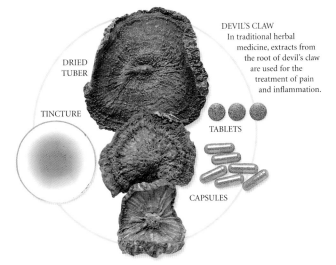

DRIED TUBER

TINCTURE

DEVIL'S CLAW
In traditional herbal medicine, extracts from the root of devil's claw are used for the treatment of pain and inflammation.

TABLETS

CAPSULES

PREPARATIONS

- ENTERICALLY COATED TABLETS

RECOMMENDED DAILY ADULT INTAKES

- 2 X 480MG TABLETS OR 15ML OF TINCTURE

PRECAUTIONS

DEVIL'S CLAW SHOULD NOT BE USED BY PREGNANT OR BREASTFEEDING WOMEN. ANYONE WITH STOMACH OR DUODENAL ULCERS SHOULD AVOID DEVIL'S CLAW AS IT STIMULATES THE PRODUCTION OF GASTRIC ACID IN THE STOMACH. IT MAY ALSO PROMOTE LOW BLOOD SUGAR AND BE UN-SUITABLE FOR DIABETES SUFFERERS.

HOW IT WORKS

Popular for hundreds of years in herbal medicine, the root of devil's claw contains substances called "iridoids," which are thought to be responsible for its action in the body. One substance in particular, called harpagoside, is believed to be especially important in helping to interfere with, and damp down, inflammatory processes.

Research has shown that devil's claw may be helpful in maintaining healthy joints, tendons, and ligaments. The anti-inflammatory effect of devil's claw has been favorably compared to prescription drugs.

THERAPEUTIC USES

● **BACKACHE**

Research has shown that two 480mg tablets of standardized devil's claw extract daily can help reduce back pain from a non-specific cause.

● **ARTHRITIS**

Tests show a potential use for devil's claw in the treatment of arthritis, lumbago, and rheumatic diseases through its ability to damp down inflammation in the body.

● **HEALTHY JOINTS**

Studies suggest that taking devil's claw supple-ments can help maintain healthy joints, tendons, and ligaments, especially in the spine and back area.

ECHINACEA

Used to prevent and treat colds and flu ● Improves skin complaints and viral and bacterial infections

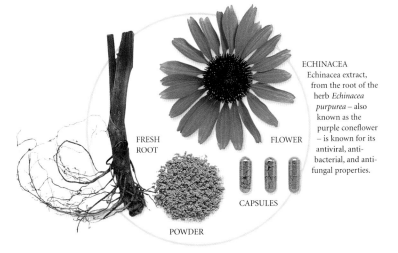

FRESH
ROOT

FLOWER

ECHINACEA
Echinacea extract, from the root of the herb *Echinacea purpurea* – also known as the purple coneflower – is known for its antiviral, anti-bacterial, and anti-fungal properties.

CAPSULES

POWDER

PREPARATIONS

- TABLETS
- TINCTURE
- CAPSULES

RECOMMENDED DAILY ADULT INTAKES

- TO FIGHT INFECTION: 2–3G, OR 15 DROPS OF TINCTURE 3 TIMES A DAY
- FOR MAINTENANCE: 1G

PRECAUTIONS

EXCESSIVE USE DURING PREGNANCY SHOULD BE AVOIDED. THOSE TAKING DRUGS TO SUPPRESS THE IMMUNE SYSTEM (E.G., FOLLOWING TRANSPLANT SURGERY) SHOULD NOT TAKE ECHINACEA. HIGH DOSES MAY CAUSE DIZZINESS AND NAUSEA.

HOW IT WORKS

Echinacea is renowned for its ability to stimulate the immune system. The substances it contains (including cichoric acid) are said to be responsible for helping to increase interferon production and improve other immune system responses. Its anti-bacterial, antiviral, and wound-healing effects may be due to the presence of "echinacin," which helps prevent the breakdown of the barrier between healthy tissues and bacteria or viruses that cause disease.

THERAPEUTIC USES

● BLADDER INFECTIONS
Echinacea is used to restore a healthy immune system and is also used to fight bladder infections.

● COLDS AND FLU
Herbalists use the herb to treat and prevent colds, flu, and ear infections. It may also help improve tinnitus – a continuous ringing sensation in the ears.

● INFECTIONS AND SKIN COMPLAINTS
Echinacea is used to treat lingering bacterial and viral infections, as well as skin complaints such as acne and skin ulcers.

● CANDIDA
Effective as a supplement or cream, echinacea appears to treat the causes of yeast and reduce the risk of re-infection.

EVENING PRIMROSE

Can help reduce the symptoms of eczema

Provides relief from pain associated with the menstrual cycle

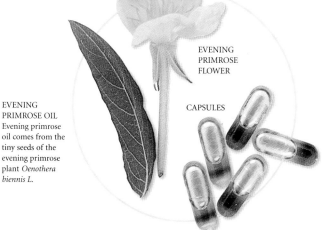

EVENING
PRIMROSE
FLOWER

CAPSULES

EVENING
PRIMROSE OIL
Evening primrose
oil comes from the
tiny seeds of the
evening primrose
plant *Oenothera
biennis L.*

PREPARATIONS

- CAPSULES
- DROPPER BOTTLES

RECOMMENDED DAILY ADULT INTAKES

- 1–3G

PRECAUTIONS

PEOPLE WHO SUFFER
FROM EPILEPSY SHOULD
AVOID TAKING EVENING
PRIMROSE OIL. IT IS BEST
TAKEN WITH FOOD TO
REDUCE THE RISK OF
NAUSEA.

HOW IT WORKS

Evening primrose oil is rich in the essential omega-6 fatty acid linoleic acid and is one of the few dietary sources of its breakdown product, gamma-linolenic acid, or "GLA." GLA is converted into hormonelike substances called "prostaglandins," which control a variety of body functions, including the regulation of hormones and the damping down of inflammatory actions.

For those people who cannot naturally convert linoleic acid into GLA, taking GLA directly as evening primrose oil supplements can have therapeutic effects on the body.

THERAPEUTIC USES

● **ECZEMA**
Evening primrose oil is available on prescription for eczema and helps to reduce inflammation, itching, and dryness.

● **HYPERACTIVITY AND DYSLEXIA**
Symptoms of both conditions have responded well to intakes of evening primrose oil and fish oils in clinical trials on children.

● **PREMENSTRUAL SYMPTOMS**
Research has shown that premenstrual symptoms of irritability, depression, clumsiness, bloating, and breast pain may improve with evening primrose oil.

FIBER SUPPLEMENT

May aid weight loss ❖ Has laxative properties

Can benefit diabetic sufferers

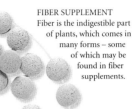

FIBER SUPPLEMENT
Fiber is the indigestible part
of plants, which comes in
many forms – some
of which may be
found in fiber
supplements.

PREPARATIONS

- GLUCOMANNAN
  KONJAC FIBER
- PSYLLIUM HUSKS
- GUAR GUM
- CHITOSAN (SEE P.92)

RECOMMENDED
DAILY ADULT INTAKES

- 18G FROM DIETARY
  SOURCES
- GLUCOMANNAN
  KONJAC FIBER:
  1–2 X 500MG CAPSULES
  AN HOUR BEFORE MEALS
- PYSLLIUM HUSKS:
  2 X 500MG CAPSULES
  WITH WATER BEFORE
  MEALS
- GUAR GUM: AS PER
  PRESCRIPTION

HOW IT WORKS

Insoluble fiber in whole-
grain food is not digested
and binds with water in
the intestinal tract. This
gives a feeling of fullness
and bulks the stools.
Insoluble fiber in fruit
and oats is gumlike and
slows the absorption of
sugar from foods.

People with swallowing
difficulties or stomach
problems should avoid all
fiber supplements.

THERAPEUTIC USES

● WEIGHT LOSS

Taken with plenty of
water, glucomannan and
psyllium husks bind with
the water in the stomach.
As a result, they give a
feeling of fullness and
reduce the desire for food
at meal times.

● CONSTIPATION

Psyllium husks have been
used for centuries by
herbalists for their laxative
properties. Today they are
used by pharmaceutical
companies in the manufac-
ture of laxative products.

● DIABETES

Research shows that guar
gum helps slow down the
absorption of sugar,
which may be helpful for
people with diabetes who
are trying to control their
blood sugar levels.

● LOWER CHOLESTEROL

Guar gum also appears
to reduce levels of
cholesterol in the body.

FISH OIL

Can help prevent further heart attack ◦ Improves symptoms of psoriasis ◦ Can benefit rheumatoid arthritis sufferers

FISH OILS
Fish oils come from the livers of white fish such as cod, or the flesh of oily fish such as salmon.

PREPARATIONS

- BOTTLED COD LIVER OIL
- CAPSULES

RECOMMENDED DAILY ADULT INTAKES

- 2–5G

PRECAUTIONS

AVOID EXCESS INTAKES OF VITAMINS A AND D FOUND IN FISH OILS. DO NOT TAKE WITH BLOOD-THINNING DRUGS, SUCH AS HEPARIN, WITHOUT A DOCTOR'S CONSENT. EPA AND DHA SHOULD BE AVOIDED BY ASPIRIN-SENSITIVE ASTHMATICS.

HOW IT WORKS

Fish oils contain the essential omega-3 fatty acid, alpha-linolenic acid, and also its derivatives, eicosapentanoic acid (EPA) and decosahexaenoic acid (DHA). EPA and DHA present in fish oil supplements help lower blood fats, thin the blood, and damp down the inflammatory processes that are involved in rheumatoid arthritis and psoriasis.

These substances are crucial for the development of an infant's brain during the last three months of pregnancy, and also for the correct development of a growing child's eyesight and sense of hearing.

THERAPEUTIC USES

● DYSLEXIA
Symptoms of both dyslexia and hyperactivity in children have improved on taking supplements containing EPA and DHA.

● PSORIASIS
Symptoms of chronic plaque psoriasis have been successfully treated both with increases in dietary oily fish such as mackerel and sardines, and with EPA and DHA supplements.

● RHEUMATOID ARTHRITIS
Fish oil supplements may reduce pain and the use of nonsteroidal anti-inflammatory drugs by people who suffer from rheumatoid arthritis.

GARLIC

May help reduce the risk of heart disease ◆ Reduces blood pressure ◆ Reduces the risk of infection and illness

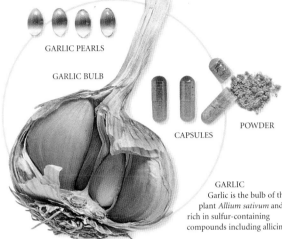

GARLIC PEARLS

GARLIC BULB

CAPSULES

POWDER

GARLIC
Garlic is the bulb of the plant *Allium sativum* and is rich in sulfur-containing compounds including allicin.

PREPARATIONS

- CAPSULES
- OIL
- TABLETS

RECOMMENDED DAILY ADULT INTAKES

- 2–3 COOKED CLOVES OF GARLIC
- 2–3 X 300MG STANDARDIZED ALLICIN-RICH TABLET, EQUIVALENT TO ½ CLOVE OF GARLIC

PRECAUTIONS

PEOPLE ON ANTI-COAGULANT DRUGS SHOULD ONLY TAKE GARLIC UNDER MEDICAL SUPERVISION.

HOW IT WORKS

Garlic is rich in sulfurous substances, one of the most important of which is allicin. Allicin is found in some, but not all, garlic supplements. It is known to help reduce "bad" LDL cholesterol in the blood, increase "good" HDL cholesterol, and lower the blood fats called triglycerides. Allicin has also been shown to reduce the stickiness of blood, especially after eating, and to lower blood pressure.

These sulfurous substances also seem to help stop the replication of bacteria acting as a natural antibiotic, and inhibit the action of both viruses and fungi.

THERAPEUTIC USES

● **HEART DISEASE**
Garlic supplements may help reduce the risk of heart disease.

● **RAISED BLOOD PRESSURE**
A reduction in blood pressure may be seen in those with hypertension.

● **INFECTIONS**
It may be possible to reduce the risk of bacterial infections and viral infections such as colds through regular use of garlic supplements.

● **CANDIDA**
Treatment of the infection candida may be possible through the regular use of garlic supplements.

GINGER

Used to treat indigestion ◈ Can improve symptoms of nausea ◈ Relieves the pain of rheumatoid arthritis

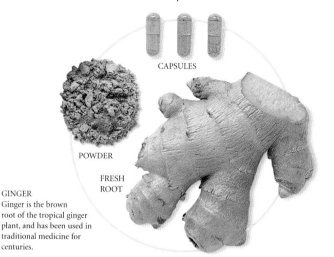

CAPSULES

POWDER

FRESH ROOT

GINGER
Ginger is the brown root of the tropical ginger plant, and has been used in traditional medicine for centuries.

PREPARATIONS

- CAPSULES
- TABLETS
- FRESH ROOT

RECOMMENDED DAILY ADULT INTAKES

- 1–2 CUPS OF GINGER TEA USING FRESH GINGER
- CAPSULES AND TABLETS AS DIRECTED

PRECAUTIONS

GINGER IS REPORTED TO HAVE BLOOD-THINNING PROPERTIES. ANYONE ON BLOOD-THINNING MEDICATION SUCH AS WARFARIN SHOULD FIRST CHECK WITH A DOCTOR. LARGE, REGULAR INTAKES SHOULD BE AVOIDED DURING PREGNANCY.

HOW IT WORKS

The key active constituents in ginger are known as oleo-resins and volatile oils, such as zingiberene. It is these substances that are thought to play a role in ginger's calming, anti-spasmodic, anti-inflam-matory, and digestive properties, as well as its ability to prevent motion sickness and the nausea associated with pregnancy.

THERAPEUTIC USES

● **RHEUMATOID ARTHRITIS**
In preliminary work on patients with rheumatoid arthritis, relief from pain and swelling was reported on a patient questionnaire after sufferers had taken

powdered ginger. Pain relief may occur through ginger's ability to reduce certain pro-inflammatory hormonelike substances called prostaglandins.

● **NAUSEA AND VERTIGO**
Ginger has been shown to improve the symptoms of vertigo and nausea, as well as morning sickness during pregnancy. It is also believed to be effective in treating nausea associated with excessive alcohol consumption.

● **INDIGESTION**
Ginger has been used in traditional medicine for thousands of years for the treatment of flatulence and indigestion.

GINKGO BILOBA

Improves mental functioning ❀ Improves body circulation ❀ Reduces the severity of asthma attacks

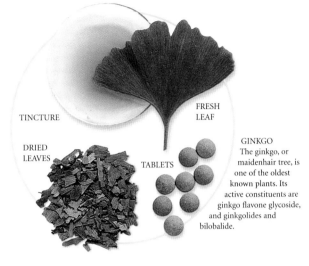

TINCTURE

FRESH LEAF

DRIED LEAVES

TABLETS

GINKGO
The ginkgo, or maidenhair tree, is one of the oldest known plants. Its active constituents are ginkgo flavone glycoside, and ginkgolides and bilobalide.

PREPARATIONS

- CAPSULES
- TABLETS

RECOMMENDED DAILY ADULT INTAKES

- 3 X 50MG TABLETS GIVING 12.5MG GINKGO FLAVONE GLYCOSIDES AND 3MG GINKGOLIDES AND BILOBALIDE

PRECAUTIONS

PREGNANT AND BREASTFEEDING WOMEN SHOULD AVOID GINKGO SUPPLEMENTS. VERY OCCASIONALLY GINKGO MAY CAUSE HEADACHES OR SKIN REACTIONS.

HOW IT WORKS

The active substances in *Ginkgo biloba* help to dilate blood vessels, allowing blood to flow freely to the legs, arms, feet, hands, and brain and deactivate potentially damaging free radicals.

THERAPEUTIC USES

● **MENTAL FUNCTIONING**
Poor concentration and memory, forgetfulness, confusion, and a reduced capacity for attentiveness can occur from a deterioration in higher mental functions brought on by aging. Improvements in the severity of these symptoms may be improved by taking ginkgo supplements.

● **SHORT-TERM MEMORY**
Tests have shown that ginkgo can help improve the short-term memory of young people.

● **PAINFUL WALKING**
Pain caused from poor circulation to the legs may be improved with ginkgo supplements.

● **ASTHMA**
Gingko appears to reduce the severity of pollen and dust-induced asthma attacks by lessening the constriction of blood vessels in the airways.

● **CIRCULATION**
Ginkgo promotes blood circulation, so may reduce the risk of conditions such as varicose veins.

GINSENG

Generates feeling of wellbeing ◆ Improves energy levels, stamina, healing, and resistance to infection

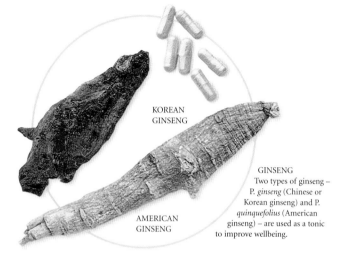

KOREAN GINSENG

AMERICAN GINSENG

GINSENG
Two types of ginseng –
P. *ginseng* (Chinese or
Korean ginseng) and P.
quinquefolius (American
ginseng) – are used as a tonic
to improve wellbeing.

PREPARATIONS

- CAPSULES
- POWDER
- LIQUID EXTRACT

RECOMMENDED DAILY ADULT INTAKES

- 2–3 CAPSULES BETWEEN MEALS
- 1 CUP OF GINSENG TEA
- 5-10G POWDER IN LIQUID

PRECAUTIONS

AVOID MORE THAN 5–10G GINSENG DAILY, TAKING AT BEDTIME, OR FOR MORE THAN 3 MONTHS CONTINUOUSLY. PEOPLE ON ANTIDEPRESSANTS NEED MEDICAL SUPER-VISION. PREGNANT AND BREASTFEEDING WOMEN SHOULD AVOID GINSENG.

HOW IT WORKS

Ginsenosides are among many active constituents in ginseng thought to be responsible for its wide-ranging benefits on the body. They are believed to be "adaptogens," with short-term effects of improving concentration, stamina, healing, resistance to stress, sexual drive, and long-term effects of wellbeing.

THERAPEUTIC USES

● ENERGY LEVELS
Limited research suggests that ginseng may help to improve energy levels.

● DIABETES
Asian ginseng has been shown to reduce blood-sugar concentrations and may, under medical supervision, be useful for those people with age-related diabetes.

● BLOOD PRESSURE
Research suggests ginseng panax may help to lower raised blood pressure.

● IMMUNE BOOSTER
Ginseng appears to stimulate the immune system of healthy people.

● HEART DISEASE
All types of ginseng may help prevent heart disease by reducing cholesterol.

● MENOPAUSE
Asian ginseng may help menopausal women suffering discomfort.

GLUCOSAMINE

Stimulates the production of connective tissue between bones ◈ May relieve pain associated with osteoarthritis

GLUCOSAMINE
Glucosamine naturally occurs in cartilage in the body and stimulates the production of connective tissue.

PREPARATIONS

• CAPSULES

RECOMMENDED DAILY ADULT INTAKES

• 3 X 500MG GLUCOSAMINE HCL CAPSULES

PRECAUTIONS

GLUCOSAMINE MAY CAUSE HEARTBURN OR NAUSEA IN SOME PEOPLE. TO AVOID SUCH SIDE-EFFECTS, GLUCOSAMINE TABLETS SHOULD BE TAKEN WITH MEALS. PEOPLE WITH DIABETES AND PEOPLE WITH WEIGHT PROBLEMS SHOULD AVOID GLUCO-SAMINE SUPPLEMENTS.

HOW IT WORKS

Cartilage is needed by the body to prevent bones from rubbing together and for absorbing shock when we walk and move. As the body ages, however, the levels of glucosamine naturally found in cartilage decrease, which may lead to reduced amounts of cartilage existing between joints. This disintegration of cartilage can lead to osteoarthritis. Taking glucosamine supplements may help the body rebuild lost cartilage and then maintain new levels into old age.

Large, long-term studies need to be carried out so the benefits and risks of taking glucosamine supplements can be investigated properly. Some early research suggests that glucosamine appears to interfere with the action of insulin and therefore may not be suitable for people with diabetes or who are overweight.

THERAPEUTIC USES

● ARTHRITIS
Long-term supplements with glucosamine may help some people to restore worn cartilage in the body and reduce both the pain and progression of osteoarthritis. For optimum benefit it may be advisable to take glucos-amine with chondroitin supplements (see also p.83).

KAVA KAVA

Relieves stress and induces feelings of relaxation ◈ May improve levels of anxiety ◈ Can help improve sleep patterns

KAVA KAVA
Standardized extracts
come from the root of
the kava kava plant –
a member of the
pepper family –
and contain active
constituents
known as
kavalactones.

PREPARATIONS

- CAPSULES
- TABLETS
- LIQUID EXTRACT
- TEA

RECOMMENDED DAILY ADULT INTAKES

- 3 X 250MG STANDARDIZED EXTRACT CAPSULES SUPPLYING 120MG KAVALACTONES EACH
- 10–20 DROPS OF EXTRACT IN LIQUID

PRECAUTIONS

AVOID KAVA KAVA IF OPERATING MACHINERY, OR TAKING DRUGS FOR INSOMNIA, PARKINSON'S DISEASE, ANXIETY, STRESS, OR IF PREGNANT OR BREASTFEEDING.

HOW IT WORKS

Kavalactone compounds in kava kava appear to act both in the brain, where they have a mildly sedative effect, and directly on the muscles, where they have a relaxant and mild anti-convulsant effect. Kava kava supplements are not intended to be taken for long-term use.

THERAPEUTIC USES

● RELAXATION

A traditional drink called sakau, made from the kava kava root, has been drunk in the South Pacific for thousands of years. It is said to bring about feelings of relaxation and wellbeing, reduce anxiety, and enhance moods.

● ANXIETY

Kava kava supplements have been found to improve feelings of anxiety, thus making the herb a potentially effective and safe alternative to prescribed antidepressants and tranquilizers for anyone suffering from various anxiety disorders.

● SLEEPNESSNESS

Taking kava kava supplements may help people to overcome periods of poor sleep patterns as the herb seems to have the ability to relax muscles and calm the mind. Taken before bedtime, kava kava may relax the body and mind, encourage sleep, and avoid the need for prescription sleeping pills.

MILK THISTLE

Repairs and protects against liver damage ✦ May help to protect the body from toxic substances

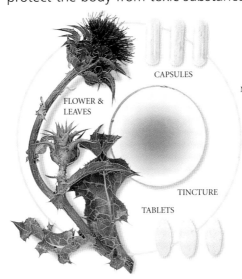

CAPSULES

FLOWER & LEAVES

MILK THISTLE Commonly found growing in North America and Europe, it is the seeds of the milk thistle plant that are used in herbal medicine.

TINCTURE

TABLETS

PREPARATIONS

- CAPSULES
- TABLETS
- TINCTURES
- BULK PREPARATIONS FOR GRINDING ONTO OR INTO FOODS

RECOMMENDED DAILY ADULT INTAKES

- 1 X STANDARDIZED EXTRACT CAPSULE OR TABLET 3 TIMES DAILY
- 10ML TINCTURE IN HOT WATER, WHICH HAS THEN BEEN COOLED

PRECAUTIONS

MILK THISTLE TINCTURE IS NOT SUITABLE FOR THOSE WITH CHRONIC LIVER PROBLEMS SUCH AS HEPATITIS OR CIRRHOSIS.

HOW IT WORKS

Milk thistle has traditionally been prescribed for protecting and repairing liver damage. Its seeds contain a compound called silymarin, which is believed to protect the liver cells from damage by free radicals, rejuvenate damaged cells, stimulate the growth of new liver cells, and generally improve the health of this vital detoxifying organ.

THERAPEUTIC USES

● CIRRHOSIS AND HEPATITIS

Milk thistle is used by herbalists to treat mild and short-term damage to the liver caused by large intakes of alcohol.

● LIVER DETOXIFICATION

Liver congestion caused by drugs such as aspirin and exposure to pollution may be improved through regular detoxification using milk thistle.

● TOXIN PROTECTION

Silymarin may block the absorption of toxins in the body, and process and eliminate toxic substances such as cadmium, carbon tetracholoride (used in dry cleaning fluids), and some wild mushrooms.

● IMMUNE SYSTEM

By increasing the liver's production of antioxidants, milk thistle may help improve the body's ability to resist infections.

PEPPERMINT

Aids digestion ❖ Can help relieve the symptoms of
irritable bowel syndrome ❖ Provides relief from nausea

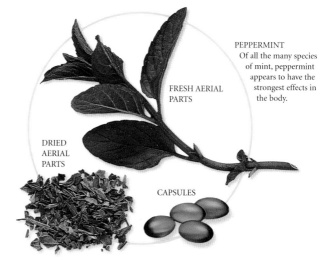

PEPPERMINT
Of all the many species
of mint, peppermint
appears to have the
strongest effects in
the body.

FRESH AERIAL
PARTS

DRIED
AERIAL
PARTS

CAPSULES

PREPARATIONS

• TEA
• CAPSULES: GELATIN &
ENTERICALLY COATED
• TINCTURE

RECOMMENDED
DAILY ADULT INTAKES

• 1 CUP OF TEA AFTER A
MEAL
• 1–2 DROPS OF TINCTURE
OR OIL IN HOT WATER
• CAPSULES AS
INSTRUCTED ON PACK

PRECAUTIONS

MINT SHOULD NOT BE
GIVEN TO CHILDREN OR
BABIES FOR MORE THAN
A WEEK AT A TIME, OR
TAKEN BY BREASTFEEDING
MOTHERS AS IT CAN
REDUCE MILK FLOW.

HOW IT WORKS

The oil in peppermint
leaves contains volatile
substances – mainly
menthol – that have
calming effects and which
help to relax muscles in
the body. Meanwhile,
other substances stimulate
the gall bladder and the
flow of bile.

THERAPEUTIC USES

● **IRRITABLE BOWEL
SYNDROME**
Research indicates that
enterically coated peppermint oil capsules, which
are not digested and
deliver the oil intact to the
colon, help to relieve the
bouts of pain associated
with irritable bowel
syndrome. They also calm

the frequency of motions
and reduce bloating.
Some of the herb's actions
appear to work through
its antispasmodic effects.

● **FLATULENCE**
Studies indicate that
peppermint can help
reduce flatulence in the
intestines and stomach.

● **GOOD DIGESTION**
The menthol in pepper-
mint increases the pro-
duction of bile in the liver
and improves its flow from
the gall bladder to the
intestine, aiding digestion.

● **NAUSEA**
Peppermint's anesthetic
effects on the stomach
wall may help relieve
feelings of nausea.

PROBIOTICS

Improves symptoms of diarrhea ◆ Provides relief from irritable bowel syndrome ◆ Improves immunity

PROBIOTICS
Probiotic bacteria can be found in food supplements and are also added to foods such as yogurt, and yogurt and fruit drinks. Probiotics include a variety of lactobaccilli and certain bifido-bacteria.

CAPSULES

LIVE YOGURT

PREPARATIONS

- CAPSULES
- TABLETS
- FORTIFIED FOOD

RECOMMENDED DAILY ADULT INTAKES

- AS DIRECTED ON CAPSULES, TABLETS, AND FORTIFIED FOODS

PRECAUTIONS

PROBIOTICS AS PART OF A DIET NEED TO BE CONSUMED ON A DAILY BASIS IN ORDER FOR THE BODY TO GAIN MAXIMUM BENEFIT.

HOW THEY WORK

Probiotics are "good" bacteria that, if ingested, have health-enhancing effects on the body. To be effective, they must survive digestion in the stomach and small intestine and progress intact to the colon to reproduce and work in different ways: outnumbering and reducing bad, "pathogenic" bacteria to give immediate beneficial effects on digestion as well as elsewhere in the body, and enhancing the immune system.

THERAPEUTIC USES

● DIARRHEA
Diarrhea as a result of antibiotic treatment and infections can be limited through the intake of *Lactobaccillus casei* and specific bifidobacteria.

● IMPROVED IMMUNITY
Certain probiotic bacteria are able to activate important parts of the body's immune system, including antibodies and macrophages, by interacting with lymph tissue in the colon.

● IRRITABLE BOWEL SYNDROME
Research work with *Lactobaccillus plantarum 299v* in fruit juice has been shown to improve symptoms of irritable bowel, significantly reducing the pain and flatulence that sufferers experience.

PROPOLIS

Can help treat colds and flu ◆ Boosts the immune system

Can help strengthen blood vessels in the gums

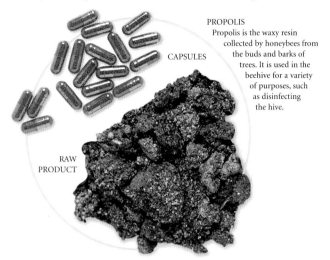

PROPOLIS
Propolis is the waxy resin collected by honeybees from the buds and barks of trees. It is used in the beehive for a variety of purposes, such as disinfecting the hive.

CAPSULES

RAW PRODUCT

PREPARATIONS

- CAPSULES
- LOZENGES
- SALVE FOR EXTERNAL USE ON WOUNDS

RECOMMENDED DAILY ADULT INTAKES

- 3 X 500MG CAPSULES
- LOZENGES TO SOOTHE SORE THROATS DURING COLDS AND INFECTIONS

PRECAUTIONS

PEOPLE WHO SUFFER FROM ASTHMA OR WHO ARE ALLERGIC TO BEE STINGS SHOULD AVOID PROPOLIS SUPPLEMENTS.

HOW IT WORKS

Propolis has a complex composition containing a huge array of flavonoids such as quercetin, vitamins and minerals, fatty acids, volatile oils, tannins, and pollen. Modern research shows that these compounds are capable of stimulating the immune system and acting as an antibacterial, anti-inflammatory, antiviral, and antioxidant in the body.

THERAPEUTIC USES

● **CANKER SORES**
Research reveals propolis to have specific antiviral effects against the herpes simplex virus, responsible for canker sores and genital herpes. Taking

propolis as soon as the symptoms of an attack occur may reduce the chances of the virus becoming a full-blown outbreak.

● **IMMUNE SYSTEM**
As people age and their immune system becomes weaker, propolis supplements may help provide plant nutrients that improve its strength and protect the body from becoming susceptible to common colds and the flu.

● **BLEEDING GUMS**
Propolis seems to help strengthen the blood vessels, particularly in the gums, where it may reduce gum disease associated with aging.

ST. JOHN'S WORT

Helps bolster the immune system ◆ Used as a safe
and efficient antidepressant ◆ Can prevent insomnia

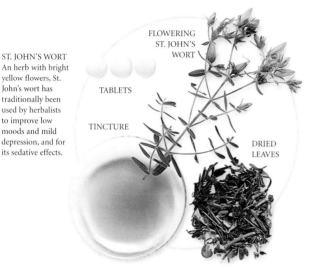

ST. JOHN'S WORT
An herb with bright
yellow flowers, St.
John's wort has
traditionally been
used by herbalists
to improve low
moods and mild
depression, and for
its sedative effects.

FLOWERING
ST. JOHN'S
WORT

TABLETS

TINCTURE

DRIED
LEAVES

PREPARATIONS

- TINCTURES
- TABLETS

RECOMMENDED DAILY ADULT INTAKES

- 3 X 250–500MG TABLETS

PRECAUTIONS

ST. JOHN'S WORT
MAY INCREASE THE
SKIN'S SENSITIVITY TO
THE SUN IN SUSCEPTIBLE
PEOPLE. IT SHOULD
NOT BE TAKEN IN
CONJUNCTION WITH
PRESCRIBED ANTI-
DEPRESSANTS EXCEPT
UNDER MEDICAL
SUPERVISION.

HOW IT WORKS

The leaves of St. John's
wort contain the substance
hypericin, which appears
to help improve levels of
"feel good" transmitters,
such as serotonin, in the
brain. It also appears to
have antibacterial effects
and to be capable of
bolstering the immune
system. It may also stop
the production of stress
hormones. St. John's wort
can also be used to treat
insomnia, gastric ulcers,
and menstrual cramps.

THERAPEUTIC USES

● MILD DEPRESSION
Studies reveal not only the
effectiveness of St. John's
wort in treating mild to
moderate depression, but

that it is also a safe and
efficient antidepressant
without the unpleasant
side effects associated
with prescription drugs.

● SLEEPNESSNESS
The calming effect of this
herb may help to correct
mild cases of insomnia.

● MENOPAUSE
Research suggests that
St. John's wort can help to
improve the moods of
women during
menopause, which in turn
can have a positive effect
on their sexual libido.

● S.A.D.
Studies suggest the herb
may reduce the symptoms
of seasonal affective
disorder syndrome.

SAW PALMETTO

Has diuretic effects ◆ Clears urinary infections
Can reduce benign swelling of the prostate gland

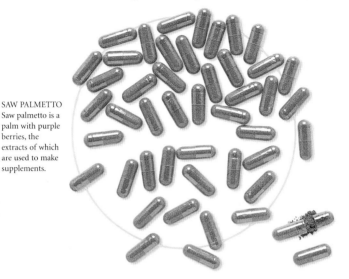

SAW PALMETTO
Saw palmetto is a
palm with purple
berries, the
extracts of which
are used to make
supplements.

PREPARATIONS

- CAPSULES
- TABLETS
- TINCTURE

RECOMMENDED DAILY ADULT INTAKES

- 2–3 CAPSULES OR
TABLETS SUPPLYING THE
EQUIVALENT OF 475MG
STANDARDIZED EXTRACT
- 2–3 X 2ML TINCTURE

PRECAUTIONS

MEN WITH PROSTATE
PROBLEMS SHOULD
CONSULT THEIR
DOCTOR PRIOR TO
SELF-TREATMENT WITH
SAW PALMETTO IN ORDER
TO RULE OUT THE RISK OF
ANY SYMPTOMS CAUSED
BY PROSTATE CANCER.

HOW IT WORKS

Active extracts of saw
palmetto berries appear
to inhibit the action of a
form of the male hormone
testosterone, reducing its
accumulation in the tissue
of the prostate gland.
Excess levels of this
"dihydrotestosterone" can
spark unwanted growth
of the gland, with
subsequent effects on the
urinary system and
urinary flow. Saw palmetto
also seems to have diuretic
effects and can have an
antiseptic effect in the
urinary system.

THERAPEUTIC USES

● **URINARY INFECTIONS**
Urinary infections may be
improved by taking
supplements of saw
palmetto, which may also
help to avoid re-infection.

● **BENIGN
PROSTATE DISEASE**
Studies have shown that
standardized saw
palmetto extract can help
both objective symptoms,
such as reducing the
frequency of nighttime
urination and poor urine
flow rate, and subjective
medical tests recorded by
a physician in those
people who have a benign
swelling of the prostate
(known as benign
prostatic hyperplasia).

SOYA

May reduce the risk of breast and prostate cancers

May reduce the risk of heart disease

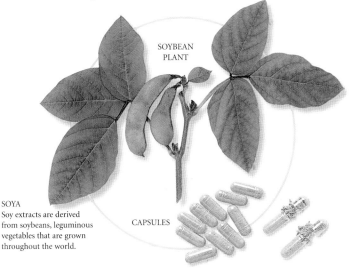

SOYBEAN PLANT

SOYA
Soy extracts are derived from soybeans, leguminous vegetables that are grown throughout the world.

CAPSULES

PREPARATIONS

- CAPSULES
- TABLETS OF STANDARDIZED SOY CONCENTRATE

RECOMMENDED DAILY ADULT INTAKES

- FOLLOW MANUFACTURERS' INSTRUCTIONS

PRECAUTIONS

IF YOUR DIET IS ALREADY RICH IN SOY-BASED FOODS, IT IS UNWISE TO TAKE SUPPLEMENTS WITHOUT CONSULTING YOUR DOCTOR FIRST.

HOW IT WORKS

Soya contains plant nutrients known as isoflavones and lignans, which have a similar structure to the hormone estrogen. When human estrogen levels are too high, these "plant estrogens" can help to damp down the effects. Lignans have an antioxidant effect, helping reduce the risk of free radical damage in the body.

THERAPEUTIC USES

● BREAST CANCER
The isoflavones called genistein and diadzein in soya appear to help inhibit the growth of cancerous cells by blocking the effect of potentially harmful levels of human estrogen.

● PROSTATE CANCER
Rates of prostate cancer are low in men who eat soya. It is possible that its "estrogenic" effects have a protective effect.

● HEART DISEASE
Regular consumption of soya has been shown to reduce levels of "bad" LDL cholesterol, which can lead to blocked arteries and heart disease. In addition to isoflavones, substances called saponins also appear to help lower the levels of cholesterol.

● HOT FLASHES
Discomfort from menopausal symptoms such as hot flashes appear to be reduced if supplements of soy isoflavones are taken.

VALERIAN

Promotes relaxation ✦ Can help establish sleep patterns

Can relieve muscle cramp

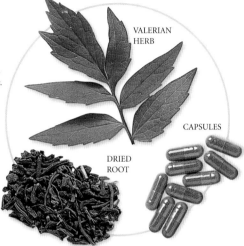

VALERIAN
HERB

VALERIAN
Valerian is the herb
Valeriana officinalis.
Its rhizome, or
root, is used to
make teas and
other herbal
remedies.

CAPSULES

DRIED
ROOT

PREPARATIONS

- CAPSULES
- TABLETS
- TEA
- TINCTURE

RECOMMENDED DAILY ADULT INTAKES

- 2–4 TABLETS OR CAPSULES CONTAINING 400MG STANDARDIZED VALERIAN EXTRACT
- 1 CUP OF TEA
- 1–2ML TINCTURE

PRECAUTIONS

VALERIAN HAS A SEDATIVE EFFECT, SO TAKE IT AT NIGHT. IT SHOULD NOT BE TAKEN WITH ALCOHOL OR OTHER SEDATIVES, OR BY PREGNANT AND BREASTFEEDING WOMEN.

HOW IT WORKS

The rhizome of the valerian plant contains "valepotriate" substances. These substances appear to have a direct effect on the brain, helping calm the nervous system and relax muscles.

It is important not to exceed manufacturers' guidance on dosage because very high doses may weaken the heartbeat. Take supplements for no more than two to three weeks to avoid the possibility of headaches and palpitations.

THERAPEUTIC USES

● STRESS AND ANXIETY
Herbalists have long used valerian for the treatment of stress and anxiety, and to promote relaxation.

● INSOMNIA
Valerian has a well-documented relaxing effect in the body and is often suggested by herbalists as a natural herbal remedy for insomnia.

● MUSCLE CRAMP
Valerian's well-known ability to relax muscles makes it of potential use for women with premenstrual muscle cramps.

VITEX AGNUS CASTUS

Improves symptoms of premenstrual syndrome

Regulates menstrual cycle ❖ Can treat acne

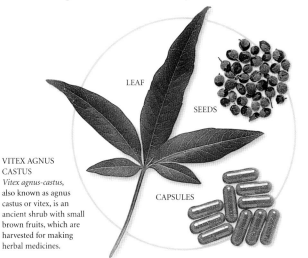

LEAF

SEEDS

CAPSULES

VITEX AGNUS CASTUS
Vitex agnus-castus, also known as agnus castus or vitex, is an ancient shrub with small brown fruits, which are harvested for making herbal medicines.

PREPARATIONS

- **STANDARDIZED EXTRACT CAPSULES AND TABLETS**
- **TINCTURE LIQUID**

RECOMMENDED DAILY ADULT INTAKES

- VITEX SHOULD BE TAKEN FIRST THING IN THE MORNING WHEN IT HAS THE GREATEST EFFECT ON THE PITUITARY GLAND. FOLLOW PACK GUIDANCE FOR DAILY INTAKE.

PRECAUTIONS

AVOID USING VITEX WHEN PREGNANT, BREAST-FEEDING, OR TAKING THE CONTRACEPTIVE PILL EXCEPT ON THE ADVICE OF A MEDICAL HERBALIST.

HOW IT WORKS

Extracts of vitex contain several active substances, including iridoids, flavanoids, and essential oil, which may work individually or together to have an effect on hormones. Known as an "adaptogen," vitex helps to normalize hormonal imbalances.

THERAPEUTIC USES

● PREMENSTRUAL SYNDROME

Clinical research has shown that vitex supplements can help relieve the bloating, breast discomfort and tenderness, nausea, cramping pain, and irritability of pre-menstrual syndrome.

● IRREGULAR MENSTRUATION

Studies suggest that vitex supplements can be helpful in regulating the menstrual cycle.

● MENOPAUSE

Vitex is used widely in Germany for the treatment of menopausal problems such as hot flashes and irritability.

● ACNE

Vitex appears to help rebalance the hormonal problems that give rise to acne, and have been reported to help improve this distressing condition.

SPECIAL NUTRITIONAL NEEDS

The nutritional needs and types of food and drink children consume changes dramatically between birth and the teenage years, as they move from a total dependence on carers for nourishment to eating independently.

BABIES

If a mother's diet is adequate, the best food for babies is breast milk. By four to six months of age a baby's body system has matured enough to introduce some solid food to supplement the milk diet, which increases the intakes of colories, protein, vitamins, and minerals, and helps develop biting, chewing, and swallowing skills.

KEY FOODS
• Infant vitamin drops may be needed if the diet of a breastfeeding mother is poor.
• Begin the six-month weaning process with small amounts of rice, vegetable, and fruit purées, then minced or mashed food, finger food, and finally chopped-up family meals.

ESSENTIAL NUTRIENTS
Breast milk supplies the correct proportion of nutrients needed by a growing baby. It also provides key immune-boosting factors to help fight infection. Modern formula feeds are an option for mothers who cannot, or prefer not to, breastfeed. Either milk should gradually be reduced to one pint a day during weaning.

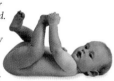

TODDLERS

This is the time to introduce as wide a range of foods as possible into the diet to avoid nutritional imbalance, establish the acceptance of a good variety of textures and flavors, and to prevent the development of fussy eating habits.

KEY FOODS
• Dairy foods or calcium-fortified soy alternatives for the development of growing bones.
• Oily fish to provide essential fats to feed a growing brain.
• Lean red meat and iron-fortified breakfast cereals to supply iron.
• A variety of fruits and vegetables for vitamins, minerals, and protective plant nutrients, and to add texture, flavor, and color.

HEALTHY ATTITUDES
Toddlers need nutritious food little and often. Too many starchy, wholegrain foods, vegetables, and fruit should not be imposed at the expense of energy-rich and protein foods. Refined, sugary, and overly fatty foods should be limited. Iron-rich foods are impor-tant to include in the diet to prevent anemia.

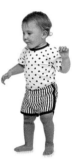

YOUNG CHILDREN

By the age of five, it is appropriate for children to be following adult guidelines for a healthy, balanced diet containing wholegrain cereal foods, five servings of fruit and vegetables a day, and lower-fat dairy alternatives. Sugary and acidic foods need to be restricted to meal times to reduce the risk of tooth decay. Should hyperactivity develop at this age, it is advisable to reduce foods containing additives – especially bright colors such as tartrazine – and try the child on a course of evening primrose oil supplements.

KEY FOODS
• Fortified breakfast cereals with milk, toast, and fruit juice make a good start to the day.
• Midmorning snacks can include a milk-based drink and fruit; main meals need to supply protein in the form of meat, poultry, fish, cheese, eggs, or legumes plus starchy foods and vegetables.
• Vegetarian children in particular may benefit from a children's vitamin and mineral supplement.

TEENAGERS

The final and dramatic growth spurts in teenage years bring with them specific nutritional needs: obtaining adequate energy; extra iron for the increased volume of blood; and plenty of calcium to support the growth of bones. Such needs must be balanced against the risk of over-eating junk foods and the risk of falling prey to eating disorders as a way of controlling and distorting normal growth.

KEY FOODS
• Dairy foods or calcium-enriched soy alternatives and iron-rich foods such as red meats are crucial.
• Wholegrain cereals, fortified breakfast cereals, oily fish, nuts, and seeds for growth and development.
• Fruit, fruit juices, and vegetables to bolster the immune system.

BALANCED APPROACH
The teenage years in particular require a balanced approach to food and the nourish-ment it provides. Teenagers who choose to become vegetarian need to pay particular attention to their dietary needs and may be advised to take a supplement supplying 100 percent of the RDA to make sure all vitamin and mineral needs are met.

CRUCIAL FOOD
Breakfast is crucial to all young children for helping them concentrate on school lessons in the morning ahead. Children can be brought up successfully as vegetarians, but may benefit from also taking a children's vitamin and mineral supplement formula.

SPECIAL NUTRITIONAL NEEDS

The nutritional needs of men and women change with age. Paying attention to different requirements and eating well throughout adult life can help protect against and treat common conditions such as heart disease and arthritis.

ADULTS

It is increasingly well-recognized that life-long health in adults, particularly men, can be improved through an appropriate diet. Heart disease, fertility, prostate problems, and stress all appear to be affected by diet. Important foods are oily fish, fruit and vegetables – especially onions and garlic – and soy-based foods such as tofu. Supplements such as saw palmetto and garlic also may be particularly useful for adult men, as may the mineral selenium.

KEY FOODS
• Mackerel, salmon, and other oily fish three times a week.
• Garlic, onions, and leeks may help to lower blood cholesterol.
• Brazil nuts, a source of selenium.

• Eat lean meat, poultry, and low-fat dairy foods and keep saturated animal fats to a minimum.

PREGNANT WOMEN

Pregnancy makes particular nutritional demands on a woman's body. Prior to pregnancy, it is advisable to take a 400mcg supplement of folic acid daily to reduce the risk of spina bifida in an infant. A diet rich in essential fats helps the development of a baby's brain during pregnancy, and means a supply is maintained through breast milk after birth.

KEY FOODS
• Folate-rich foods such as Brussels sprouts, beets, and fortified breakfast cereals.

PROTECTING YOUR HEALTH
Achieving and maintaining the correct weight for height plays a significant role in protecting not just the cardiovascular system but the joints and back, reducing the risk of degenerative diseases such as stroke and arthritis.

NUTRITIOUS DIET
A healthy diet during and between pregnancies helps a mother maintain and replenish her stores of vitamins and minerals. This is especially important in non-meat eaters, who may also benefit from taking supplements.

• Oily fish like salmon, mackerel, and sardines for essential fats.
• Red meat, leafy vegetables, nuts, seeds, and legumes to provide iron.

POSTMENOPAUSAL WOMEN

The maintenance of women's health after menopause can be helped enormously by diet. Improving food sources of plant estrogens and antioxidant vitamins and minerals may help to slow both visible signs of aging and the hidden risks of aging in women, which are associated with reduced levels of estrogen – including osteoporosis and heart disease.

KEY FOODS
• Soy-based foods such as tofu, soy milks and yogurts, and soybeans, which provide plant estrogens.
• Dairy products and calcium-enriched foods such as fruit juices and some breakfast cereals.
• A wide range of fruits and vegetables, especially berries and citrus fruits, which may help to reduce visible signs of aging of the skin while also protecting the eyes and maintaining good vision.

STAYING HEALTHY
As the metabolism slows with increasing age, body weight becomes an issue for many postmenopausal women. Regular physical activity and sensible, healthy eating guidelines can help to stabilize weight at a desired level and help improve not just physical health, but self esteem and psychological wellbeing.

THE ELDERLY

It is well recognized that the process of aging both affects nutritional needs and is affected by the nutritional composition of the diet. While long-established good eating habits can help reduce the risk of certain cancers and heart disease in later life, health can be optimized with good dietary practices at this stage. Memory, eyesight, mobility, and overcoming the drain on nutrients caused by some drugs may make supplements a valuable part of an elderly person's diet.

KEY FOODS
• Red meat and canned oily fish complete with bones for particularly good sources of well-digested and absorbed iron and calcium.
• Bananas and fruit juices for increased potassium to maintain mental clarity and antioxidants to fight cataracts, glaucoma, arthritis, and mental degeneration.
• Multivitamin and mineral, garlic, gingko, and fish oil supplements may be appropriate if advised by a doctor.

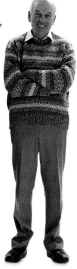

MAXIMUM BENEFITS
The aging process reduces the absorption of some nutrients, and appetites tend to be smaller, so the smaller quantities of foods consumed must be well-balanced. Eating to maximize the immune system, reduce inflammatory conditions such as arthritis, and keep the bones strong is crucial.

READY RECKONER

If you have a medical problem, it is vital that you first seek professional medical advice. With your doctor's consent, it may be possible to help certain common ailments with vitamin, mineral, or herbal supplements.

CONDITION	HELPFUL SUPPLEMENTS	TIP/ADVICE
COLDS Caused by viral infections that lead to inflammation in the linings of the nose and throat. Sore throats, sniffing, sneezing, a runny nose, and headaches are well-recognized symptoms of the common cold.	Limited research suggests that supplementing with four 500mg intakes daily of vitamin C may reduce the severity of cold symptoms and improve recovery times. Zinc lozenges may relieve a sore throat, and garlic and echinacea appear to help the immune system to fight infection.	High intakes of vitamin C may lead to diarrhea and an acid stomach in susceptible people. If this is the case, try non-acidic versions of the vitamin, such as ester-c. When reducing vitamin C mega-doses such as these, do so slowly to avoid withdrawal symptoms and scurvy.
PMS Occurring around ten days prior to menstruation, the symptoms of pre-menstrual syndrome can include mood swings, breast tender-ness, headaches, water retention, low energy levels, and irritability. Symptoms can vary from mild to severe.	While not consistently effective in clinical research, some women find that vitamin B6 supplements improve the symptoms. Evening primrose oil has been proven effective in treating premenstrual breast tenderness, bloating, and irritability, while magnesium may also be beneficial.	In tests using standardized evening primrose oil, women with premenstrual syndrome were given six 500mg capsules daily to build up levels of its active component GLA. Lower intakes of poor-quality evening primrose oil may not be adequate to elicit an effect.

CONDITION	HELPFUL SUPPLEMENTS	TIP/ADVICE
OSTEOPOROSIS Leading literally to a thinning of the bones, osteoporosis is caused when minerals such as phosphorus and calcium are removed from the structure of bones more rapidly than they are replaced. This results in weakened bones and the risk of fracture.	Daily intakes of 1,000mg of calcium may reduce the risk of bone fractures, and particularly help those on dairy-free diets. Vitamin D is crucial for calcium absorption, so to aid absorption 10mcg of vitamin D daily may be useful, as well as fish oil and evening primrose oil.	Avoid rhubarb, which reduces calcium absorption. For maximum deposition on the bones, take calcium supplements in the evening. Regular exercise also helps the body to replace lost calcium in bones.
INFERTILITY Defined as the inability to conceive a child after one year of regular, unprotected intercourse, infertility affects one in six couples at some time. Where male fertility is the problem, supplements may be helpful.	Male smokers may benefit from 250–1,000mg a day of vitamin C to improve sperm counts; 600mg a day of vitamin E may help men with low sperm levels. Beta-carotene may help sperm maturation, and daily zinc supplements could benefit sperm mobility.	For both partners, it is useful to pursue recreational activities that help you to relax and unwind, since stress can play a role in fertility problems. Taking yoga or relaxation classes may also be helpful.
ECZEMA An inflammation of the skin – accompanied by itchiness, redness, and sometimes scales and scabs – is distressing to those affected. While it may result from a number of underlying factors, including stress and allergies to chemical irritants, diet may also play a role.	The Efamol evening primrose oil supplement has been proven in clinical trials to improve the itchiness and redness associated with eczema. The GLA it contains helps to form hormone-like substances called prostaglandins, which can damp down skin inflammation.	In some cases, eczema begins to clear if milk, dairy products, and eggs are removed from the diet. Harsh detergents are best avoided, and stress may be tackled with relaxation techniques such as yoga. Two drops of lavender oil in the bathwater may also help.

CONDITION	HELPFUL SUPPLEMENTS	TIP/ADVICE
PSORIASIS An inflammatory skin disease, which results in thick, red patches covered by a silvery scale. Psoriasis particularly affects the elbows, knees, scalp, torso, and back. In some cases, the affected areas can become infected.	Fish oil supplements of 3g daily have been shown to improve symptoms as the EPA present in the oil helps to damp down inflammation. Intakes of 15mg of zinc daily and 250mg of vitamin C may help the body fight infection within the psoriasis plaques.	Drink an infusion three times a day of burdock root and water (simmered for 15 minutes) to improve scaly skin. Increase intakes of oily fish such as salmon, mackerel, and sardines, and cut back on saturated animal fats in your diet.
POOR CONCENTRATION AND TIREDNESS An inability to concentrate and constant tiredness can be symptoms of full-blown and sub-anemia, caused through poor iron intakes. Non-meat eaters are particularly at risk, especially teenage girls and women. Symptoms can affect everything from school-work to driving skills.	A multivitamin and mineral supplement with 15mg of iron a day can help to replenish dietary deficiencies. Choose a supplement that also provides the correct RDA for vitamin C, copper, and the B-vitamin folic acid, which all assist iron absorption.	Avoid taking supplements with tea because the tannin inhibits the absorption of iron. Be careful not to take extra zinc above the RDA as it reduces the availability of iron to the body. If meat is not part of your diet, include oily fish, the dark meat of turkey and chicken, nuts, and seeds in your diet.
LOW MOODS Low moods and mild depression can lead to a pervasive feeling of sadness, which affects people in different ways. Symptoms include intense misery, negativity and self-doubt, tearfulness, crying, insomnia, and loss of appetite.	Clinical research has proven that standardized extracts of St. John's wort are as effective as prescription drugs in helping to relieve these symptoms. Valerian, which aids relaxation and promotes good sleep, may also be useful.	Try to share your feelings and avoid long periods alone. If symptoms persist, medical advice should be sought. Clary sage essential oil is a powerful relaxant and helps to lift moods: place 2–3 drops in a bowl of steaming water and then inhale.

CONDITION	HELPFUL SUPPLEMENTS	TIP/ADVICE
BACKACHE Backache, such as a slipped disk or a nerve or muscle injury, can be painful and debilitating. Once medical opinion has ruled out specific causes, it may be possible to find relief with herbal supplements.	Research indicates that a standardized extract of devil's claw may help treat nonspecific back pain. Vitamins and minerals that help reduce inflammation, such as evening primrose oil and fish oil, may help.	Massage, exercise, and relaxation tips can help improve symptoms. If overweight, gradual and steady weight loss to achieve a normal weight can be one of the most effective strategies for relieving back pain.
INSOMNIA Difficulty in getting to sleep or staying asleep is often caused by anxiety, but may also stem from illness, pain, lack of exercise, depression, or noise pollution.	Valerian and passiflora can aid sleep, as can combined supplements containing relaxant herbs such as *Melissa officinalis*, extract of hops, and lemon balm.	Gentle exercise, lavender oil in a bath, and relaxation techniques before bedtime can help. Avoid caffeinated drinks such as tea and coffee toward the end of the day.
RAISED CHOLESTEROL High cholesterol can lead to atherosclerosis (the deposition of fatty layers on artery walls), resulting in clogged arteries, restricted blood flow, and increased risk of heart disease.	Standardized extracts of garlic may lower raised cholesterol levels. Fish oil supplements containing EPA appear to reduce levels of blood fats and thin the blood to lessen the chance of blood clots.	Avoid saturated fats in butter, cream, full-fat dairy foods, and fatty meat and meat products. Achieving a normal body weight and regular gentle exercise can also lower cholesterol levels.
IRRITABLE BOWEL SYNDROME A condition affecting the colon, which can lead to diarrhea and/or constipation, bloating, pain, and cramps, IBS is often of unknown cause, but can affect physical and psychological health.	Peppermint supplements reduce gas and bloating. Probiotic supplements restore good bacteria in the colon and may help to alleviate symptoms. Evening primrose oil and fish oil mixes can reduce inflammation.	Eat probiotic foods such as live yogurt. In some cases, excluding wheat from the diet or increasing fiber relieves symptoms, while other people respond well to relaxation techniques such as meditation.

GLOSSARY

ALPHA-TOCOPHEROL: Type of vitamin E that accounts for 90 percent of the vitamin in human tissue.

ANGINA: Sense of constriction and pain that often radiates down the arms, resulting from a lack of blood to the heart.

ANTHOCYANINS: Violet, red, and blue water-soluble antioxidant pigments in fruits, berries, flowers, and leaves.

ANTIOXIDANTS: Substances that help protect against potentially damaging free radicals in the environment.

BACTERIA: A group of micro-organisms, some of which benefit the body and others that cause disease.

BETACAROTENE: An orange/yellow pigment in plants (which is masked by the green pigment chlorophyll in vegetables such as spinach).

BIOFLAVONOIDS: Also called flavanoids, these are a group of over 2,000 pigments in plants that have strong antioxidant functions and give plants their color.

CAPILLARY: A tiny, thin-walled blood vessel forming part of a large network of vessels. They allow the rapid exchange of substances between fluids and surrounding tissue.

CARCINOGENIC: Cancer-causing agents.

CHOLESTEROL: Found in all body tissue, cholesterol is essential for many metabolic functions. It is carried, bound to proteins, in the blood. Too much of the low-density protein lipoprotein is a risk factor for heart disease.

DAIDZIEN: A type of isoflavone in soybeans, tofu, and soy milk.

DIABETES: A condition characterized by raised blood sugar due to a deficiency, lack, or diminished effect of the hormone insulin.

ENZYME: A type of protein that acts as a catalyst for various reactions in the body.

ELLAGIC ACID: A phenolic flavanoid with antioxidant properties.

ESTROGEN: A generic term referring to hormones released from the ovaries. These include estriol, estrone, and estradiol.

FREE RADICALS: Unstable, reactive substances formed in the body as a result of natural respiratory processes and in response to triggers such as exposure to ultra-violet light, smoke, and air pollution. Free radicals are constantly being made and broken down. They are thought to have the potential to damage cells in the body, which in turn can be the starting point for some diseases such as cancer and coronary heart disease.

GLAUCOMA: A condition where the intraocular (the inside of the eye) pressure is raised.

GLUTEN: The protein complex in wheat or rye.

GLYCEMIC INDEX: This index of foods is simply a ranking of foods based on their immediate effect on blood sugar levels.

HOMOCYSTEINE: Made in the body through the rapid conversion of the amino acid methionine, homocysteine carries out rapid repair work on surrounding tissues and is then quickly converted back into methionine. This process requires the B vitamin folate.

HORMONES: Specific chemical substances secreted by endocrine glands and carried in the blood to regulate the function of tissues and organs elsewhere in the body.

INSULIN: A hormone made in the pancreas that is secreted into the blood and removes excess blood sugar to maintain constant levels. People with diabetes may require injections of insulin.

ISOFLAVONES: Plant nutrients that are found in soy and soy products, and have mild estrogenlike effects in the body.

LIGNANS: Plant nutrients found in flaxseeds, berries, and wholegrains, which have antioxidant and oestrogenic effects in the body.

MACULAR DEGENERATION: Degeneration of the macula lute, the yellow spot on the retina of the eye that is the area of clearest vision. This eye condition is the most common form of age-related blindness.

PROSTAGLANDINS: Substances secreted by a range of body tissues. Their production can be influenced by dietary intakes.

PSORIASIS: A chronic skin disease of red areas covered with scales.

RETINOIC ACID: A substance derived from retinol (vitamin A), used in the treatment of acne.

RDA: Recommended daily (or dietary) allowance or (amount).

STANDARDIZED EXTRACT: An extract of an herb that contains a set concentration of the active substance.

TANNIN: Found in tea, carob beans, and unripe fruit, tannins give an astringent effect once in the mouth. Tannin binds with some nutrients such as iron, making it unavailable for the body to digest.

TINCTURE: A mix of alcohol and water into which a herb's active components dissolve.

ZEAXANTHIN: A carotenoid with antioxidant properties and yellow pigmentation, found in corn and egg yolk, for example.

ACKNOWLEDGEMENTS

AUTHOR'S ACKNOWLEDGEMENTS: I would like to say a very hearty thank you to my editor Susannah Steel, who has made the writing of this book a pleasure, and to Alison Lotinga who organized the wonderful artwork. Thank you also to MC and Daphne at Dorling Kindersley for your continuing support.

DK WOULD LIKE TO THANK: Sarah Ashun, Paul Bricknell, Jonathan Buckley, Andy Crawford, Michael Dent, Phillip Dowell, Mike Dunning, Andreas Einsiedel, Neil Fletcher, Steve Gorton, Barnabas Kindersley, Dave King, David Murray, Ian O'Leary, Stephen Oliver, Roger Phillips, Susanna Price, Tim Ridley, Jules Selmes, Karl Shone, Clive Streeter/Patrick Mcleary, Matthew Ward, Jerry Young for photography. Denise O'Brien, Melanie Simmonds, Marcus Scott at the DK Picture Library. Hilary Bird for the index, Maggi McCormick for American text changes. Sharon Flynn at Holland & Barrett Retail Ltd for supplying supplements.

CREDITS: p.18: peppermint & capsules – Judith Smallwood; p.110 raw product of Propolis – Bee Health Limited.